C0-CCN-717

FEMALE ENDURANCE ATHLETES

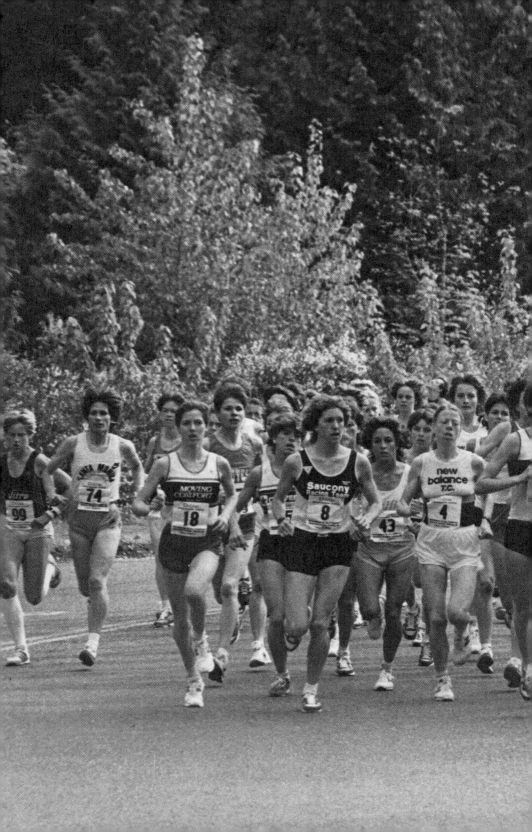

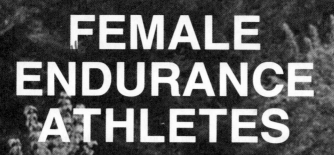

FEMALE
ENDURANCE
ATHLETES

Barbara L. Drinkwater, PhD
Pacific Medical Center
Seattle, Washington

Human Kinetics Publishers, Inc.
Champaign, Illinois

Library of Congress Cataloging-in-Publication Data
Main entry under title:

Female endurance athletes.

Proceedings from a conference held at Olympia, Washington in May 1984.
Includes bibliographies and index.
1. Women athletes—Physiology—Congresses.
2. Marathon running—Physiological aspects—Congresses.
3. Endurance sports—Physiological aspects—Congresses.
I. Drinkwater, Barbara L., 1926-   . [DNLM:
1. Physical Endurance—congresses. 2. Physical
Fitness—congresses. 3. Sports Medicine—congresses.
4. Women—congresses. QT 255 F329 1984]
RC1218.W65F46 1986   612'.044   85-30243
ISBN 0-87322-043-9

Developmental Editor: Susan Wilmoth, PhD
Production Director: Ernie Noa
Copy Editor: Terry Jopke
Text Layout: Cyndy Barnes
Interior Design: Julie Szamocki
Cover Design and Layout: Jack Davis
Printed by: Braun-Brumfield

ISBN: 0-87322-043-9

Copyright © 1986 by Barbara L. Drinkwater

Printed in the United States of America

10 9 8 7 6 5 4 3 2 1

Human Kinetics Publishers, Inc.
Box 5076, Champaign, IL 61820

Acknowledgments

The Scientific Congress was made possible by the generous contributions of the sponsors and the efforts of the Thurston County Women-Can-Do Committee. Special thanks are due to Denise Keegan who conceived the idea of "Women in Sports: From Athens to Olympia," a special prerace program of events that included the Scientific Congress.

CONFERENCE SPONSORS:

Safeco Life Insurance Company of America

Washington State Beef Commission

The Weyerhaeuser Company

The Forrest Foundation

Tree Top, Inc.

The Evergreen State College, Olympia

J.C. Penney

South Sound Center, Lacey

Hospital Corporation of America (Black Hills Community Hospital, Olympia)

Producer of the Conference:

Thurston County Women-Can-Do Committee

Contents

Preface

The U.S. Women's Olympic Trials Marathon held on May 12, 1984 in Olympia, Washington was a historic first for women runners. Although prohibited from running any race longer than 800 m until the 1960s and barred from official participation in the marathon event until 1970, women runners in the late 1970s were campaigning vigorously for the right to run the 26.2 mile distance in the 1980 Olympics. The stumbling blocks to their success were a lingering concern that women were physiologically unsuited for endurance events and the need to satisfy the Olympic requirement that competition in an event be available in 25 countries on two continents before it can be an Olympic sport. As late as 1980, leaders of the International Amateur Athletic Federation were still focusing on physiological issues in denying a request to include a women's marathon in the 1984 games.

It would be nice to record that research scientists were responsible for debunking the myths inhibiting women from achieving their potential as endurance athletes, but the credit must go to the athletes themselves. The women who persisted in running longer distances in spite of rules, ridicule, and even physical restraint proved by example that women could run the marathon. They, in turn, provided a subject pool for scientists interested in studying how such strenuous and prolonged exertion affects the female athlete. Many of the misconceptions regarding women as endurance athletes had come from studies using sedentary or moderately active women as subjects. For the first time, scientists could focus their research skills on superbly conditioned and highly motivated women.

The results of their studies have appeared in professional journals over the years but have never been brought together in one publication. When the Thurston County Women-Can-Do Committee decided to include a Scientific Congress among the prerace events, they provided a perfect opportunity to bring together many of the scientists who have contributed to our understanding of the female endurance athlete. Because this occasion celebrated women's achievements as athletes, it seemed particularly fitting to invite as speakers many of the women who supplied the basic scientific data supporting women's efforts to run an Olympic marathon.

The Proceedings include two chapters that were not presented at the Congress because of time constraints but are an important aspect of the total picture. No one can really appreciate the achievement of the women who ran in Olympia without knowing the events leading up to that historic day. Joan Hult's paper provides that perspective. Karen Nilson's chapter on injuries to female runners is particularly appropriate in light of Joan Benoit's victory in the trials marathon just 17 days after arthroscopic surgery on her right knee. Both authors kindly accepted an invitation to enlarge the scope of these Proceedings by contributing a chapter in their special area of interest.

Jackie Puhl examines three factors vital to endurance performance—body composition, muscle characteristics, and energy supply—and how biological sex differences in these variables may affect performance. Dorothy Harris summarizes the psychological data specific to women runners and discusses how running affects a woman's psychological well-being. It is apparent from Betty Atwater's paper that there is still much to be done to add to our knowledge of how biomechanical factors relate to the performance of female runners and even to their potential for injury. Emily Haymes covers an area of great interest to all athletes which is of even greater concern for women runners, whose desire to maintain minimal body fat often conflicts with adequate nutrition. Dr. Haymes also addresses the problem of iron deficiency among female runners and discusses the value of iron supplementation.

Everyone recognizes that the marathon is a grueling event which places exceptional demands on the human body. Very few runners understand how that stress is reflected by changes in blood chemistry. Christine Wells and her colleagues describe the changes they observed in a group of male and female runners following the Fiesta Bowl Marathon and discuss the interpretation of these deviations from the normal state. Dr. Wells mentions the effect of hyperthermia on blood chemistry, and in the following chapter, I summarize the often conflicting data regarding male and female response to thermal stress. Because one of the most frequent arguments against women running distance events was their supposed intolerance to heat stress, it is reassuring to report that female runners are at no greater risk than males when running in the heat.

The irregularity or cessation of menses, the so-called athletic amenorrhea experienced by some female endurance athletes, is addressed by Charlotte Sanborn. After reviewing the various hypotheses regarding its etiology, she discusses the latest research linking the hypoestrogenic state with a decrease in bone density in the amenorrheic athlete.

As women continue to compete in the marathon, sport scientists will continue to do research on varying aspects of their performance. May both groups be applauded for their efforts and may the female endurance athlete go on to reach her highest potential.

Barbara L. Drinkwater, Editor

1 The Female American Runner: A Modern Quest for Visibility

Joan S. Hult
University of Maryland

The revival of the modern Olympics in 1896 heralded a new struggle against excluding women from the Olympic Games. As the Games were to open in Athens, a Greek woman, Melpomene, secretly trained to compete in the marathon despite the refusal of Olympic officials to sanction her entry. Pierre de Coubertin, the French founder of the modern Olympics, had made the Games a male preserve, declaring it "neither fitting nor proper that women should perform in public."[1] Nevertheless, Melpomene chose to run beside the official runners from Marathon to Athens, finishing in 4-1/2 hrs. Despite substantiation by journalists and bicycle followers that she successfully completed the marathon route, her achievement went unrecognized.[2] Thus, Melpomene was the first "invisible" female marathon runner. Eighty-eight years later in the Los Angeles Olympics of 1984, American runner Joan Benoit emerged from the Los Angeles Coliseum tunnel to the cheers of more than 100,000 spectators and became the first gold medalist in an Olympic Marathon for women, with a time that would have won 11 of the 20 men's Olympic Marathons (2:24:52). Benoit's is a milestone in a series of achievements by elite female athletes to overcome lack of encouragement and recognition, cultural disapproval, absence of a sport tradition, lack of training and "mentoring," hostility on the part of the physical education establishment, and in some cases actual denial of competitive opportunity by the Olympic leadership.

Acknowledgment is gratefully given to Paula Dee Welch for her extensive research on women in the Olympics and Jacqueline Hansen and Joe Henderson for their assistance on women in long-distance running. The author is indebted to Rosalie Gershon for her work as editorial consultant and to Carol Jackson for her technical assistance.

In conducting the research, extensive use was made of the archives of the National Association for Girls and Women's Sports housed at American Alliance for Health, Physical Education, Recreation and Dance (Reston, Virginia). Unless otherwise noted, all manuscript material cited is from these archives. The archival collection of the Amateur Athletic Union (Indianapolis, Indiana) also proved to be helpful. Unpublished manuscripts by Joan S. Hult are available from her.

This work examines the female struggle for equal opportunity by viewing her role, nature, function, and conflicts as social patterns and appropriate sport behavior changed for the modern female athlete in general and for the runner in particular. Changes over time are studied within the historical/social context and in two major settings, education and popular culture. The three epochs treated are: (a) 1880 to 1920; (b) 1920 to 1950; and (c) 1950 to the present. This study recognizes gender as a fundamental variable within sport history. Further, visibility in this paper is defined as official recognition. Thus, behavioral norms and social patterns are inextricably bound with the female athlete's fight against exclusion from world class competition. As George Eliot rightly observed, "There is no private life that has not been determined by a wider public life."

Historical Perspectives

Before discussing the struggle of the modern female athlete for elite competitive experience, it is appropriate to observe women's participation in sports throughout history and within different cultures. As with history in general, women's history has been perceived and recorded from the male historian's perspective, and much information has either been lost or was never recorded. In a definitive 2nd century A.D. study of Greek athletics by Pausanias, for example, an observation regarding female participants in the Heraean Games was that "Their hair hangs down, a tunic reaches to a little above the knee, and they bare their right shoulder as far as the breast."[3] Such treatment is comparable to the modern description of swimmers in terms of their costume rather than their prowess. When George Orwell wrote in 1939 of the "invisibility" of the peasant class in the British Colonial Empire, he spoke of the allegiance to their own of the power-holders within a society and their ability to see as heroic or meaningful only those representing a mirror image of themselves:

> The people have brown faces—besides, there are so many of them! Are they really the same flesh as yourself? Do they even have names? Or are they merely a kind of undifferentiated brown stuff, about as individual as bees or coral insects?[4]

Ancient Women Athletes

Women participated in athletics in the ancient societies of Egypt, Crete, Greece, and Rome; some even had names. While women were denied participation in the sacred festival to honor Zeus (the Olympic Games) and under penalty of death were also barred from being spectators, this does not mean that sports did not exist for women in ancient times. The aforementioned women as well as women from Asia Minor participated in ball games, swimming, chariot racing, acrobatics, equestrianism, and footraces.[5] Egyptian and Cretan women added wrestling to their sporting lives, and a few Roman women were gladiators.[6]

The affluent Egyptian women participated in an astonishing number of ball games, ritualistic dances, and cultic footraces, in part as a testimony of their ability to rule. The depiction, for example, of Queen Hatshepsut running a cultic footrace is found among the artifacts of the Egyptian civilization. Similarly, the women of the Minoan society in Crete had cultic footraces to demonstrate their physical prowess. An activity unique to the women of Crete was the sport of bull grappling, in which they competed alongside the men as toreadors (perhaps the first coed team sport).[7]

According to Eisen in his thesis on *Sports and Women in Antiquety*, ". . . vase painting, sculptures, and literary records testify to the popularity of running and footraces among women in Greece." He also notes that evidence of swimming, chariot racing, and wrestling have been found among the artifacts and inscriptions. Among the Greek city-states, the Spartan women enjoyed the greatest variety of sporting events. They dominated female contests, no matter what the event, because they alone had been prepared to be warriors. Their training programs were designed to develop physical perfection, albeit for an ulterior motive—the reproduction of male offspring. Nevertheless, their physical prowess in footraces, swimming, and combat sports is legendary.[8]

The ancient women had their own version of the Olympic Games, designed to honor Hera, the wife of Zeus. The games took place in the Olympic stadium the year preceding the more prestigious Olympic Games. The only event in the Heraean Games was the footraces, conducted for three different age-groups running a distance of about 168 yards, or 5/6 of the men's "Stade Race." The winner of each age-group received the traditional olive leaves for her prize, a portion of the beef sacrificed to Hera, and an opportunity to have a statue erected in the temple of Hera or in her hometown. The figurine of a Spartan youth in the Vatican Museum and the bronze statue in the British Museum attest to the presence of women and the honor bestowed on young female footrace winners. There is also some evidence that well-established contests for women athletes were held in the same cities as those for men; that is, in the Panhellenic games of Olympia, Nemean, Isthmia, and Delta as well as other local contests. There were female athletes from other than the Greek mainland, suggesting the games were sizable events.[9] Yet the actual artifacts are few in number, leaving the modern world to speculate about the accomplishments of the "invisible" female runners.

Greek mythology clearly defines footraces and sports such as equestrianism, hunting, and shooting as accomplishments of some of the early goddesses. Greek long-distance running was aptly symbolized by the greatest runner, male or female, in the mythical world, Atalanta. According to legend, Atalanta (strong, capable, beautiful), certain of her fleetness of foot, offered

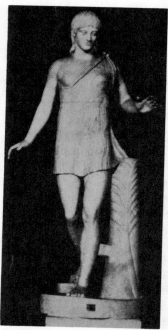

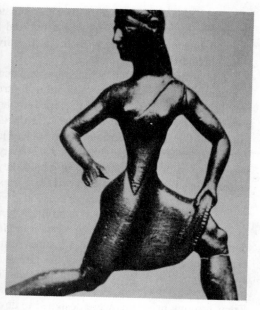

Figure 2   "Spartan Athlete in Heraia Races at Olympia."
Bronze Figurine depicting a female Spartan athlete in the
Spring. London British Museum. *Note.* From *The Eternal
Olympics (The Art and History of Sport)*, by Nicolaos
Yalouris (Ed.), 1979, New Rochelle, New York: Caratzas
Brothers.

Figure 1   "Statue of Girl Runner,"
Vatican Museum. Copy of Fifth
Century original from a photograph
from Alinari. *Note.* From *Greek
Athletic Sports and Festivals,* (p.
49) by E. Gardiner, MacMillan
and Co.: London, Reprint from
Wm. Brown Company. In the
Physical Education Series.
Dubuque: Iowa.

to marry any man who could defeat her (and put to death those who tried and
could not). She met her downfall when Melanion succeeded in distracting her
with three golden apples during their race; while she picked up the apples,
he won.[10]

American Women Before 1880

Women in early American history, like their counterparts in ancient times,
suffered from invisibility. Before 1820, American women often participated
equally in the work required to sustain home and family. Thus, a certain amount
of physical prowess was essential. *The Journal* of Sarah Kemble Knight (1704
to 1705) for example, reflects the rigorous lifestyle of an independent-spirited
wife and mother traveling along the East Coast over rough roads, where she
crossed perilous rivers, traveled long distances on horseback, and visited

dangerous inns. Her description of a harrowing experience crossing a river in an unsafe canoe accentuates her ability to cope.[11]

As the center of the American economy and productivity moved to the marketplace, women no longer shared the work in the same way. Their work was increasingly performed at home, while their husbands' was done in the marketplace. As the patterns changed and distinct, separate roles were assumed by each sex, a European Victorian model emerged. This model, with its confinement of women to domestic tasks at home, completed the polarization of the sex roles. The personality traits, social responsibilities, and behavior patterns attributed to these separate roles evolved throughout the 1820 to 1880 era, and the roots of masculinity and femininity were firmly interwoven into the fabric of American life by the 1880s.

"The Cult of True Womanhood," a Victorian concept, was characterized by the pale, docile, nurturing and submissive woman who was placed on a pedestal to be admired. She was given some freedom to be a "lady of leisure," partly as evidence of her husband's affluence and social status. As the family's guardian of morality, she was held responsible for the ethical mores of her children and even of her husband. In addition, her religious training required obedience to her husband and acceptance of her own subordinate condition.

Masculinity, conversely, was defined by success in the marketplace, the presence of a "lady of leisure" at home, and social interaction with other men within the sporting tradition. Men saw the world in Darwinian "survival-of-the-fittest" terms, with "rugged individualism" providing the rationale for action in the "real" world of their own making.

The period 1820 to 1880 was one of social and religious reform, with the major movements—abolition of slavery, public education, and health reform—affecting everyone. Other reforms, however, were given impetus by women. Women's concerns such as reform of prisons, sanitariums, hospitals, and mental institutions attempted to provide the basis for a more egalitarian society. The joining together of women in these reform movements provided a forum for increasing expectations and lent an urban and political ambiance to the suffrage movement and the birth of the "new woman" of the 1880s to 1920s.

Women in Sport Before 1880

Sport opportunities were available on a class-stratified basis. Affluent women were encouraged to pursue simple recreational activities such as crochet, archery, crew, walking, swimming ("bathing"), and a few outdoor activities such as hunting, fishing, and fox hunting.[12] The rise of the middle class and of organized sport led some women to attempt previously all-male sports such as horseracing and equestrianism and many more to participate in professional pedestrianism (a walk-run race). More prominent activities, however, for all classes included (even with clothing restrictions) ice skating, roller skating, and sledding. Health reformers such as Catharine Beecher promoted correct diet, exercise, and mild forms of recreational activities. Calisthenics and gymnastics became popular in the women's colleges.[13]

The foremost journal for women, *The Godey's Lady's Magazine*, expressed the etiquette of sport and set the boundaries of sporting endeavors. The journal supported recreational pastimes, while discouraging vigorous sporting activities. However, despite these efforts, many women wanted sport experiences and sought them in the popular culture.[14]

A few bold women moved outside the security of their cultural sex roles to experiment with activities such as being circus trainers and participating in horse racing, cycle racing, and pedestrianism. One of the earliest accounts of a women's pedestrian race was recorded in the *Spirit of the Times*, April, 1832, but the pedestrian race generally occurred in conjunction with the men's event and was a rarity until after the Civil War. Thereafter, increased interest and prize money resulted in men and women having separate as well as some mixed contests. Having events for both men and women brought larger crowds than did the separate contests and there were often thousands of spectators at the course's end.[15]

A typical event for women only was a pedestrian race in which 50 miles were to be covered in less than 12 hours. On April 27, 1877, for example, Miss Mary Marshall, the "Champion Lady Pedestrienne of the world" would attempt the "extraordinary feat of 50 miles inside of 12 hours." The hours were to be from 10 a.m. and if successful would finish at 10 p.m. Admission was 50 cents with a purse of $50.[16] A greater but less-frequent feat, however, occurred in the ladies' six-day go-as-you-please walking contests in which the ladies covered between 350 and 390 miles, yielding a purse as high as $975. The prize money was provided by the sponsors and spectators' admission fees. Another form of pedestrianism was women competing in long-distance contests. Early in 1879, "Madame Anderson walked 2,700 quarter miles in 2,700 hours on a track set up in Mozart Gardens in Brooklyn. Soon afterward, however, Madame Exil de la Chapelle covered 3,000 quarter miles in 3,000 hours in Chicago." "The *National Police Gazette* depicted ladies as 'glamorous, attractive, buxom beauties,' and described the affairs from the erotic viewpoint, rather than as athletic," according to John Cumming, author of *Runners and Walkers: A Nineteenth Century Sports Chronicle.*[17] As men moved away from professional pedestrianism to amateur track-and-field meets, the sport died; women's pedestrianism suffered the same fate.

Summary

Thus, at the dawn of the Modern Age in 1880, many patterns were already set, and others that would influence sport had begun to emerge: the separation of men's and women's worlds into two separate cultures, the latter of which was characterized by recreation rather than competitive sports; the beginnings of the health reform and exercise movements, which later served to "permit"

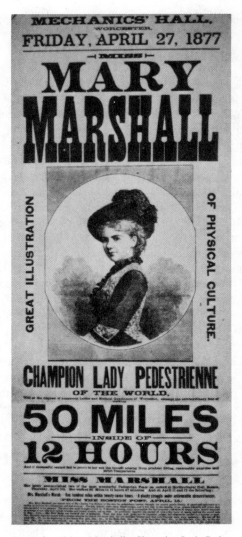

Figure 3   "Mary Marshall—Champion Lady Pedes-
trienne—American Antiquarian Society." *Note.* From
*Runners and Walkers: A Nineteenth Century Sports
Chronicle* (p. 102). By John Cumming, 1981,
Chicago, IL: Regnery Gateway.

women to evade the "Cult of True Womanhood" with a physiological/medical
rationale; the placement of large numbers of women within the educational
system; and the participation of a few bold female role models in traditionally
"masculine" activities such as horse racing and pedestrianism. Sport for some
was beginning to provide a way to escape the narrow intellectual and spiritual

confinement based on gender difference and to promote the pursuit of a new self-image.

1880-1920

The "New Woman" in American society of the 1880s and 1890s had begun to function apart from her limited domestic role, enjoying greater independence and wider professional choices. In so doing, women encountered an entrenched, culturally-induced sport tradition that systematically excluded women and whose purpose was to initiate young men into rigidly defined gender identification. This "Rite of Passage" vis-a-vis sport has proven to be a theme of undeniable influence on athletics for girls and women.

The "Rite of Passage" of this era has its roots in ancient civilizations, but it is more formally expressed in the late 19th and early 20th centuries through the works of such men as educator and play reformer G. Stanley Hall and playground movement leaders Luther Gulick and Clark Hetherington. The political leader, Theodore Roosevelt, led the crusade to reestablish the American sense of national purpose and manifest destiny through the rejuvenation of the male population through sport. Sport was thus used to reaffirm patriotic-military loyalties in a less dangerous arena and provide a testing ground for the sex role socialization process. Given these aims, what place might girls and women have in sport? Certainly not strenuous, competitive physical activity.[18]

Sports were seen as a useful means for training young males to deal with the pressures of urban life and lessening ethnic conflict within the "melting pot." Further, sports were seen as beneficial in changing the prevailing perceptions of male and female sex roles by incorporating the feminine trait of morality within the masculine psyche. Thus sport furthered the goal of sportsmanship and character development; the ideal "team player" would become the ideal male citizen.[19]

Because the public schools were attended by girls as well as boys (and sometimes in greater numbers, since boys sometimes had to drop out to find work), there was a need for a female sport environment to inculcate the values of the team sport experience as it applied to women. Therefore, it came about that within the educational setting, physical education was used primarily to teach girls the values of health and social interaction and only incidentally character building or high-level competition.

The educational system during this era, 1880 to 1920, established the direction of physical activity for girls and women. In the new sport tradition, role-appropriate individual sports for girls and women were the elite, nonviolent sports played by gentlemen, such as tennis, golf, archery, yachting, and crew. Mass (common) sports such as track and field and bowling were thus not considered appropriate for women. Similarly, sex-appropriate team sports for women were either those in which men did not compete, such as field hockey, or those modified by women for female participation, such as basketball and volleyball. By these class and gender-based criteria, softball was not an acceptable sport for girls. Track and field, including long-distance running, was considered an activity acceptable perhaps in a recreational setting, but not within the competitive environment. For example, when a Ms. Ballintine, a teacher at Vassar College, promoted a field day for all Vassar women in the Spring of 1895 (the first such competitive event for women on the collegiate level, and perhaps in any setting), she was severely criticized for conducting a sport inappropriate for the college woman.[20]

By the last two decades of the 19th century, women's sphere of interest was changing. In an *Atlantic Monthly* article, the "transitional American woman" was seen as one who had found occupation, respectability, and even dignity apart from the home.[21] Educational curricula began to shift from the domestic sciences, nursing, and teaching to a wider variety of offerings, and a trend toward liberal arts education was begun. While marriage was still the norm between 1860 and 1900, in two generations nearly 10% of the female population would remain single. These same "bachelor girls," as they were called, would move in large numbers to more vigorous outdoor activities, such as hiking, mountain climbing, bicycling, canoeing, fishing, swimming, and a few in tennis and golf.[22]

Two independently-occurring phenomena—the clothing reform and the bicycling mania—interacted with and influenced each other. The happy result was that by the end of the 1890s, women were able to shed the costuming of the past and feel a new independence of movement and spirit.[23] Women might no longer be strapped up like hourglasses in clothing such as corsets and long skirts that were, as Frances Willard phrased it "absurd to the eye and unendurable to the understanding." The early leaders of the feminist movement such as Amelia Bloomer wore that first vestment of women's liberation named for her, the "bloomer." It was not, however, until women discovered the excitement of the bicycle that clothes reform took on new meaning to the sportswoman. The bicycle offered independence in travel, companionship as an equal for boyfriends outdoors, and a cure for the depression of "cabin fever." Willard joyously explains the influence of the bicycle on women:

> The old fables, myths and follies associated with the idea of women's incompetence to handle bat and oar, bridle and rein, and at least the crossbar of the bicycle, are passing into contempt in presence of the nimbleness, agility, and skill of 'that boy's sister.' Indeed, if she continues to improve after the fashion of the last decade, her physical achievement will be such that it will become the pride of many a ruddy youth to be known as 'that girl's brother.'[24]

Although it is interesting to read of the achievement of bicycle racers and the distances that some women covered (e.g., 17,152 miles in one year), the freedom and the introduction to the world of sport it gave to the average woman is more important.[25]

Educational Domain

Meanwhile, on the college campus, the prevalent insistence of many medical experts on feminine physical and emotional frailty had a negative effect on public acceptance of female scholars. Too much exposure to the rigors of the academic world, they warned, might lead to abnormal reproductive functions.[26] Now, decades later, it can be seen that women in general accepted this concept of frailty partially because they respected medical authority (in the absence of conclusive scientific data), and also perhaps because the concept fit so neatly into the desired gender behavior set found in "The Cult of True Womanhood." Claiming frailty allowed working women some escape from the long hours in the garment trade or in the shop. The concept of feminine emotionality was also promoted by commercial enterprises such as manufacturers of health tonics for women. *Lydia E. Pinkham's Private Textbook Upon Ailments Peculiar to Women* gives this advice:

> The mother of any girl who is passing through this monthly disturbance [menstruation] should be very careful to guard her in every possible way. . . . Intense mental excitement should be avoided, the extremes of merriment or anger, laborious study or brain activity of any kind or alike matters which may cause great injury.[27]

Physical educators attempted to strike a delicate balance between encouraging vigorous physical activity and condemning roughness and masculine behavior that causes "women to do sadly unwomanly things." The gymnastic drills of former days were replaced in the second decade of the 20th century with sports, including the vigorous team sports and track and field events, although high jumping and pole vaulting soon lost favor, and the events were confined to those considered appropriate for women. Women continued to participate in the sports of the previous two decades, but greater emphasis was placed on the team sports of basketball, volleyball, and field hockey. Senda Berenson, in her defense of basketball, commented in the 1901 edition of the *Basket Ball Rules for Women*:

> Now that the woman's sphere of usefulness is constantly widening, . . . now that all fields of labor and all professions are opening their doors to her, she needs more than ever the physical strength to meet these ever-increasing demands . . . Games are invaluable for women in that they bring out just these elements that women find necessary today in their enlarged field of activities. Basketball is the game above all others that has proved the greatest value to them.[28]

By the second decade of the 20th century, track-and-field events had won favor within the Eastern women's colleges and Midwest colleges. There is also ample evidence of competitions for women in track and field before the 1920s. High schools in small towns often held track and field meets for girls as well as for boys, with some state championships for girls before the end of the era. This suggests the tremendous change in attitudes toward vigorous sports for girls and women.[29]

While many physical educators still argued against jumping events as dangerous to the health and welfare of the student, the use of such events in recreational settings earned the approval of many women physical educators and large numbers of men. Independent groups permitted different kinds of races for girls in recreational settings while the boys were in track meets. Although the first national championship in track and field did not occur until 1923, the Amateur Athletic Union (AAU) discussed the possibility of track for girls and women at about the same time they were discussing the issue of competitive swimming, as early as 1916.[30] Articles in the *American Physical Education Review* by Dr. Harry Stewart in 1914 and again in 1916 encouraged the use of track events for all female high school and college students.[31]

Popular Culture

Commercialization of leisure had its effect among working class women as large numbers attended public amusements such as dance halls, amusement parks, variety theaters, and movie houses. Comparatively few of this large group participated in the sporting activities of the middle class, although some saw the need for healthy physical activity and tried bowling, bicycling, water sports, and the out-of-doors winter sports. The next generation of women joined company teams, industrial leagues, company-sponsored basketball competition, track-and-field teams, bowling leagues, and summer softball. The playground movement and settlement houses encouraged girls and women in such sports even in this era, thus opening the door for some working class women to experiment with such sports as track and field and to move toward some forms of competitive meets.[32]

Within the popular culture, the highlight of the first decade of the 20th century for tracksters was the 1903 Madison Square Garden Physical Culture Exhibition in which prizes of solid gold watches were given to each of the winners of five different track events. The 50-, 220-, 440-, and 880-yard events were used, and the finale was a mile run.[33]

AAU and Olympic Movement

Even before 1920 American women were entering world-class competition. During the epoch under discussion, American women competed only in the sex-appropriate sports (tennis, figure skating, golf, archery, and swimming) in the Olympics, and these despite the fact that De Coubertin continued to proselyte for an all-male Olympics:

> The Olympic Games represent the solid period of manifestation
> of male sports based on internationalism on loyalty as a means,
> on art as a background and the applause of women as a
> recompense.[34]

Although France and America voted against including women's swimming events in the 1912 Olympics, by 1916 the AAU decided to field a team despite its earlier opposition. This was a significant breakthrough for female athletes. Although thwarted by the suspension of the Games during World War I, in 1920 the United States fielded a full swimming contingent. This helped establish a precedent, so that although track and field was not considered a sex-appropriate sport, the door had been set ajar for seeking approval for entry into the women's 1922 Olympics in Paris.[35]

The first official recognition of the extent of amateur female track participation occurred at the 1916 AAU convention, which voted to keep records of women in swimming and track and field. It is, however, clear from sport literature that opportunities were available even before World War I.[36]

Summary

As women entered the Golden Age of Sport in the 1920s, they had found that the first cause of invisibility was themselves. They had taken the first step toward visibility by looking in the mirror and finding an independent image rather than the reflected view of a husband or family. Further, while the question of sex-appropriate sports was to haunt female participants for decades, the barriers to the sport experience itself were ready to fall. In her search for some form of highly competitive sport experiences, the educator's egalitarian cry for universal participation in the Golden Age of Sport would eventually have an overwhelming effect on women's opportunity to participate in sports.

1920-1950

After World War I, America's growing economic and political power ushered in an era of prosperity and optimism that shaped many areas of American life in the 1920s that had strong implications for the world of sport. The mobility of the population, more leisure time, and relaxation of the restrictive standards created a climate that favored greater opportunities for women in many spheres of life. Victory at the ballot box (19th Amendment; 1919) encouraged women to take advantage of their new independence. The public schools, which now reached most Americans, provided physical education and thereby the beginnings of sporting experiences for girls. The Golden Age of Sport for men became a miniature Golden Age of Sport for women.

The years under discussion, 1920 to 1950, were particularly significant in the development of women's sports. Seen in perspective, the 1920s provided the growth and proliferation of a variety of sports (including those of the middle and working classes). The education setting saw the beginnings of an experimental female model of athletics that was based on the ideal of universal participation and that differed significantly from the male model of athletics.

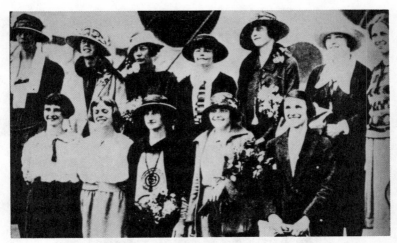

Figure 4   "American Team to Women's Olympics in Paris." *Note*. From *Track and Field Athletics for Girls*, 1923, New York: American Sports Publishing Co.

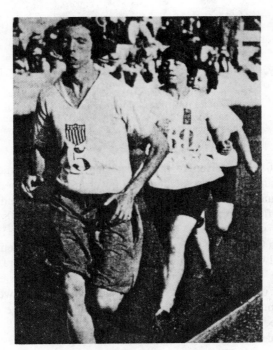

Figure 5   "Women's Olympics—Paris, 1922." *Note*. From *Track and Field Athletics for Girls*, 1923, New York: American Sports Publishing Co.

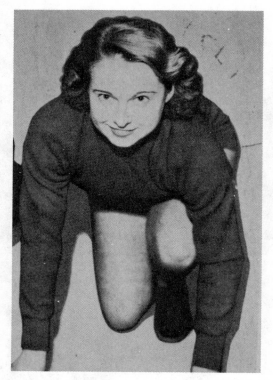

Figure 6   "Betty Robinson—1928 Olympics." *Note.* Photo courtesy of the American Olympic Commitee, *Report of the American Olympic Commitee,* 1928, New York: American Olympic Commitee.

The 1930s, the period of the Great Depression, saw the building of government-supported sport facilities and government-sponsored programs in recreational and competitive sports, including those for girls and women. The media's glorified portrayal of women role models of the 1920s led to public acceptance of skilled athletes. Role models included Gertrude Ederle, Helen Wells, Glenna Collett, and Babe Didrickson. An image of the youthful, healthy American girl was extolled in the women's magazines of the era.[37] The 1930s also saw the fruition of the influence of the female physical education establishment in the form of play days and sport days. This slowed the growth of varsity sport and led highly competitive athletics to move underground (outside the educational domain).

The decade of the 1940s was pivotal in changing the attitudes and behavior patterns of women. The war years demanded strong, healthy workers in the labor market to replace the men at war. Competition became one means to develop "fitness for war" in programs sponsored or encouraged by the federal government.[39]

The 1940s also gave women physical educators experience in conducting highly competitive sport programs for the War Department and in leading some elite caliber activities for the armed services. This experience later challenged athletes to question their provincial attitudes. Finally, by the end of the 1940s, the separate interests of the physical educators, amateur athletic establishment, and popular culture had merged to forge a supportive environment for highly competitive sports. In short, the 1920 to 1950 period that gave rise to organized sport for women was one of great intellectual and philosophical ferment, larger-than-life heroes, significant medical studies, and vast organizational achievements.

Educational Domain

The formation of a United States track-and-field team to compete in Paris in 1922 was the catalyst in 1923 for the new Women's Division of the National Amateur Athletic Federation (NAAF) to join its sister organization, the Committee on Women's Athletics (CWA)* of the American Physical Education Association (APEA) to protest the participation of women in the Women's Olympics.[40] It was not, to paraphrase Shakespeare's Caesar, that they loved elite athletics less but that they loved the ideal of universal participation more. The National Section on Women's Athletics (NSWA) member during the 1920s and 1930s would be quick to point out that the organizations were not against competition but merely against the wrong kind of competition; namely, varsity or elite athletics at the expense of sport for the majority of girls and women. They were concerned with the financial drain on educational institutions and physical education personnel if called on to provide both athletics for the masses *and* special, time-consuming training for the limited number of elite (Olympic) athletes. Thus, physical educators chose to expend their energies developing new individual and team sports for the ever-increasing number of high school and college students.[41]

The overriding result was a greater participation base, which benefited the average woman, who was then equipped to maintain a sport interest for health and recreation. As Agnes Wayman put it:

> Do we want to have a nation of girls who participate in sports because they love them? Do we believe in a democracy of sport

---

*The Committee on Women's Athletics became: Women's Athletic Section (1927-1931); National Section on Women's Athletics (1932 to 1953); National Section for Girls and Women's Sports (1953 to 1957); Division for Girls and Women in Sport (1957 to 1974); National Association for Girls and Women in Sport (1974 to the present). These organizations are substructures of American Physical Education Association (1903 to 1937); American Association for Health, Physical Education and Recreation (1938 to 1974); American Alliance for Health, Physical Education and Recreation (1974 to 1979); American Alliance for Health, Physical Education, Recreation and Dance (1979 to the present). The Association for Intercollegiate Athletics for Women (1971 to 1979) was a substructure of DGWS/NAGWS before becoming an independent association in 1979. These initials will be used in the text of this paper.

based on that attitude? Or are we going to lend our influence toward
an aristocracy of sport based on superiority of skill?[42]

The underlying political belief here is egalitarian. Its referent is "the
greatest good for the greatest number"—"a sport for every girl; every girl
in a sport." The philosophical concept of equality among sports offered in
the program also reflects this democratic theme. Sport programs for girls within
the educational system encouraged all sports from archery to volleyball. By
contrast, sport for boys and men had developed a major-minor emphasis with
football and basketball at the top of the social hierarchy, thereby implying that
some sports were considered inferior to others. (Track and field held a lower
position in the male hierarchy.)

The health and welfare of the participant was paramount in the minds of
the women's leadership. They feared that the male model of athletics with its
emphasis on the spectacle, the "winning syndrome," and commercialism would
infect the newly-developing female sport tradition. In a female model of
athletics, physical educators wished to protect the health and safety of the participant, and this included considerable concern that rough sports would be
detrimental to child-bearing. A final concern was for the possible loss of the
"feminine" psyche in gladiatorial combat.[43] By the 1940s many of these myths
that had thwarted elite competitors were dispelled by medicoscientific research.
The myths that disruption of the menstrual cycle had a harmful effect on child
bearing or that athletic performance must be curtailed during menstruation were
simply disproved. The research indicated that healthy women accustomed to
activity might safely pursue sport any time; that is, they should not be regard-
ed as having an "unnatural delicacy."[44] Further, the idea of psychological
damage from too much emotional stress lost favor in view of the evidence.
This shift in attitude was significant in the changing patterns of competitive
athletics in the post-war years.

According to Agnes Wayman, the physical education establishment held
a philosophical belief in female self-determination in athletic governance and
values:

> Our ideals and standards have been set by men. What is sauce for
> the gander is *not* sauce for the goose. . . . Men took the tiller—
> they offered us the tow, and we, forgetting that we are a frail craft,
> as to speak, took it. . . . We are setting forth under our sail manning
> the whole craft.[45]

To control the "craft," however, women physical educators saw a need
to control women's athletics. In order to do so, they set out to develop new
leaders in teaching, coaching, and officiating, who would be "steeped" in
the sport traditions of the NSWA. This was certainly a maternalistic approach
to setting standards and establishing guidelines for conducting sporting
experiences for women. They were convinced it would assure that the traditional
views of physical educators would be perpetuated. The women believed that
only women could understand the psychological, motivational, and physio-

logical needs of the female. There was concern that the male model of athletics could creep into the women's programs unless it was carefully guarded against.[46]

The outcome of this philosophy within the educational realm was the cessation of competitive athletics in favor of the less competitive play days in which events involving other institutions required mixing different schools' teams to avoid school loyalties and combat. A few outspoken physical educators were frustrated by the absence of the competitive edge. As Ina Gittings said in 1931:

> Play for play's sake. What does this mean? . . . I picture the girls
> in a play day as sheep huddled and bleating in their little play
> meadow, whereas they should be young mustangs exultantly racing
> together across vast prairies.[47]

It is a misconception, however, to believe there was a complete burial of varsity or elite competition in educational institutions. Examination of new primary source material indicates instead that the play day was truly triumphant only during perhaps the 1925 to 1950 period and in urban rather than rural areas. Further, community, amateur, and industrial competition flourished. In fact, nonschool programs grew to such an extent that by the 1940s the physical educators were forced to concede that women were looking outside the educational setting and finding considerable opportunity for competition.[48]

In spite of the curtailment of varsity programs, there were interscholastic and intercollegiate athletics in this period, but they were somewhat invisible to the women leaders. The women physical educators did not discourage the individual and upper class sports (tennis, golf, figure skating, and swimming) as much as the sports for the masses. The invisible sports forced underground (basketball, track and field and softball) emerged stronger than ever in the industrial leagues, AAU, and in small schools. The will to find competitive opportunities surfaced even in the absence of any long sport tradition and despite the social taboos against such participation.[49]

In keeping with the NSWA's philosophical commitment to the principle of women controlling women's athletics, there developed a power struggle between the women's physical education leadership and the AAU over the desirability of competitive athletics and the control of athletics for women. The philosophical reasons behind the clash have been described earlier. As a result of their opposition to varsity and elite sport, the women's organizations actively protested the 1922 Women's Olympic Games and the track-and-field events in the 1928 Games, and they withheld their support for the 1932 and 1936 Olympics.[50] Since the AAU was the primary organization sending athletes to the Olympics, conflict arose between the AAU and the NSWA. Another reason for the conflict was the absence of leadership positions for women within the AAU until the appointment of Dee Boeckmann (the U.S. entry in the 800-meter race in the 1928 Games) to the Basketball Committee in 1934. She subsequently became a track-and-field coach in the 1936 Olympics and head of the Women's Division of Track and Field.[51] Conversely, the AAU wanted the NSWA's support to increase the prestige of their events and the number of volunteer workers and to provide more opportunities for competitive experiences for the female athlete.

Because the AAU preferred cooperative interactions with the women's groups they made numerous overtures to obtain their support. When the questions of control and leadership arose, and AAU made some rudimentary efforts to enlist women into local coaching and leadership positions, but they showed less enthusiasm for having women in prestigious decision-making roles. In answer to the problem of female leadership, AAU formed a 16-member Women's Advisory Committee and selected women to officiate a notable women's track-and-field meet at Madison Square Garden in 1933.[52] As mentioned earlier, they selected Dee Boeckmann for the basketball and the track-and-field positions. The AAU/NSWA conflict had the long-term effect of moving more of women's athletics outside education and into the public sector.

After World War II, competition for female athletes took on a new meaning, and the controversy surrounding what was appropriate for women shifted toward acceptance of competitive athletics. Women physical education leaders moved toward a procompetition stand which incorporated the "pyramid concept" in physical education; that is, instructional classes followed by intramurals and then perhaps varsity athletics. The concept of a structure for competitive athletics was even discussed at professional meetings. In addition, the NSWA moved out to the larger amateur athletic sphere and recognized that they had to surrender some of their opposition to and control of elite competition in order to accommodate the new attitudes and behaviors of female athletes.[53]

Popular Culture

The kinds of sports in which upper-class women participated expanded as more of these women refused to be excluded from some of the traditional male strongholds. Increasing numbers invaded sports such as polo, lacrosse, motor racing, harness racing, shooting, and mountain climbing. The traditional elite sports for women remained popular as the sporting experiences of the upper- and middle-class women continued to expand. Sports outside those considered to be "sex appropriate" were the responsibility of organizations and industrial business enterprises that sponsored competitive leagues. The AAU became the most important organization that sponsored women's swimming, basketball, volleyball, and track-and-field competitions from local to international levels. It is within the AAU structure and its position in the Olympic movement that the understanding of the role and the conflicts for the distance runners can best be understood. Throughout the epoch, female athletes were experiencing greater opportunities within industrial programs, recreational and church programs, and in private clubs. Public sport organizations, including those from the playgrounds, settlement houses, and

YWCA programs, were gradually increasing the sport offerings for girls and women.[54]

AAU and Olympic Movement

The prelude to the AAU's entry into the field of women's track and field occurred as a result of a modern Heraean festival called the Paris Women's Olympics of 1922 (Ladies International Track and Field Meet). The prime mover of the event was Madame Alice Milliat of France, who had formed the Federation Sportive Feminine Internationale, world governing body of women's track and field. Through the organization Madame Milliat had asked the International Olympic governing body to include track and field events for women. Upon refusal by the officials she organized the first Women's Olympic Games in 1922 (first International Women's Games). The events were held in 1922, 1926, 1930, and 1934. By the 1934 games, there were 11 events with 200 athletes from 17 countries, and more than 15,000 spectators attended.[55] Despite disapproval from the physical educators, the American athletes took part in all four of the Games. Following the "takeover" by the International Amateur Athletic Federation (IAAF) of women's track and after the Games of 1934, the demise of the Federation was imminent.

The AAU began its attempt to control women's athletics when Dr. Harry Stewart boldly announced in June 1922:

> The International Federation of Women Athletes was formed in Paris. They are to hold an international meeting in August of 1922 and America hopes to have a team . . . further he states, let the girl have the joy of competitive athletics under proper restrictions and develop to the utmost her physical powers, every one of which will be of unestimable value to her in the complexities of modern life.[56]

In January 1923, the AAU voted to have women register for all sports within their jurisdiction: swimming, gymnastics, and handball. They rejected "any desire to control women's boxing, weight lifting, wrestling, tug-of-war, and water polo."[57]

The first national championship in track and field took place in Newark, New Jersey, in September 1923. Most of the competitors were from the East Coast and were sponsored by industry or business establishments such as banks or insurance companies (such as the winner, Prudential Life Insurance), and a few teams represented private track clubs. In future years, recreational centers and towns would also sponsor track teams. The championship was reported to have been "well patronized by competitors and spectators with very commendatory statements from them." Yet the leaders admitted that some "militant few persist in condemning such competition entirely."[58]

In an effort to create a truly national championship, the AAU accepted an offer from the Pasadena Athletic and Country Club to conduct the 1925 nationals and to provide $2,000 to bring "stellar" athletes from the East and

Midwest to the nationals.[59] By the end of the 1920s more than 900 competitors gathered in Chicago to compete in the nationals, while as many as 4,000 screaming Chicagoans cheered the runners. The 1930s brought ever-increasing numbers to the nationals to provide a larger pool of athletes for selection on the Olympic teams. In addition, high school championships were still a reality in spite of the antivarsity sentiment. A 1923 and 1927 report claimed teams and championships in widely separate areas of the country, such as New Jersey, St. Louis, Chicago, and southern California.[60]

In the meantime, behind the scenes in the Olympic movement in 1926 the American AAU contingent tried to promote a full program of track-and-field events for women at the 1928 Games. They cited the success of the AAU nationals as evidence of the desire, need, and importance of track-and-field events for women.[61] Despite their efforts, the IAAF voted to permit only five events to replace the 11 of the Women's International Games, but their action was a start in the right direction.[62]

In the 1928 Games in Amsterdam, for the first time female track athletes were permitted to perform and perspire within the sacred arena of the Olympics. The lone American victor was a 16-year old, Betty Robinson, who became the first American woman to receive a gold medal in a track-and-field event. (She also won a medal in the 1936 Games, but missed the 1932 Games because of an injury.)[63]

The infamous 800-meter disaster for the female distance runners was a marvelous opportunity for the opponents of women in track to echo, "I told you so." No journalist did it as dramatically or as often as John Tunis (1929), who expressed his point of view in *Harper's* a few months after the Olympics:

> Below on the cinder path were eleven wretched women, five of whom dropped out before the finish, while five collapsed after reaching the tape. I was informed later that the remaining starter fainted in the dressing room shortly afterward.[64]

Consequently, after the Games of 1928 the Olympic Congress of 1930 spent an entire day discussing the women's competition, including the possible removal of all track-and-field events from the 1932 Games. The 1928 Games were "experimental," they argued, and the experiment had not worked. The American delegates, among the strongest advocates of the women's track events, threatened to boycott the men's track events if women's events were not retained. This power play was successful—women's track and field remained in the Olympics—without, however, the 800-meter run, which was eliminated until the 1960 Olympics.[65]

The years following the triumph of having women's track and field in the Olympics and then Babe Didrikson's 1932 Games were not as buoyantly hopeful as many had expected. In 1928 the presidency of the AAU went to Avery Brundage. He was not very sympathetic to the cause of women's sports. While his public posture was not harmful during the early years in office, by the end of the 1932 Olympics he became an outspoken ally of the antiwomen's Olympic movement, particularly in track and field. After the 1936 Games, Brundage commented on being fed up with women as track-and-field competitors, suggesting ". . . her charms sink to something less than zero. As swimmers and divers, girls are beautiful and adroit, as they are ineffective and unpleasing on the track."[66]

Fortunately for track and field, his views were not shared by a majority of the committee for the 1936 Games. A motion to eliminate women's track-and-field events was defeated by a slim 11-9 vote to maintain track.[67]

Summary

By midcentury, then, the rise of sport for women was complete. An experimental model of athletics had been articulated and effectuated in the educational domain. Sports also flourished in the popular culture (i.e., the realm where the powerful AAU held control), and in diverse community and industrial leagues. In retrospect, the post-World War I years seem buoyant and somewhat innocent in spirit, since female role models such as Eleanora Sears, Babe Didrikson, Gertrude Ederle, and Eleanor Holm were pioneers and pacesetters by virtue of their competitive spirit. They were iconoclastic and often feisty. Their journey was largely isolated, unshared, and unshareable to a world that had not caught up to them. Today, elite women athletes have support and a ready-made sport structure. The female athletes of the first half of the century had their whole being challenged; they met that challenge in a way that has somewhat smoothed the same rugged pathway for the next generation of athletes.

1950-Present

The large number of women undertaking new roles and responsibilities during World War II, particularly in the industrial labor force, returned to home life with a sense of achievement—and nowhere to use their new skills. Only as the postwar economy began to expand the job market could women discover new perspectives, options, and self-images.

The publication of Betty Friedan's *The Feminine Mystique* rekindled the feminist light of the suffragists in the form of the "women's liberation movement."[68] Federal legislation supporting equal pay and equal employment opportunity, the Civil Rights Act, the Equal Rights Amendments, the use of the 14th Amendment in judicial lawsuits, and Title IX of the Education Amendment of 1972 all contributed to a strongly felt need to move toward equity in the sporting tradition. The women's liberation movement also contributed two major psychological effects to the sports tradition for women: (a) a belief among female sport participants that their own needs, rather than those of family or boyfriends, were acceptable; and (b) a spirit of group cohesion ("bonding") that built on the female model of athletics' cooperative ethic.

Women were beginning to have time, motivation, and opportunity to participate in one form or another in the sport experience. Against the backdrop of the wider labor market, women had a reason to finish high school and attend college. They were often the first in their family to attend college. These women, of course, were ripe targets for the goal of the physical educators: "a sport for every girl, every girl in a sport." The educators tried to encourage their students to continue recreational sport throughout their lives.

With this burgeoning of athletic and recreational opportunities, the educational sport leadership found that it could no longer function as the guardian of traditional values for girls and women in sport. While many emerging leaders had been schooled in the concepts and practice of play days and sports days, the new freedom for women and their own wartime experience with competitive programs brought a new attitude and desire to help their female students achieve a higher level of athletic excellence.

The protest of the Olympic Games became history for the new breed of women leaders within the DGWS/NAGWS. The growing restlessness of skilled female athletes made apparent a need for new directions for highly skilled athletes within and outside of the educational domain. Women were going to compete in sports offered in the popular culture and were seeking out highly competitive programs for their newfound skill. Nonschool athletic programs under the sponsorship of the AAU expanded to include more local, regional, and national championships in track and field.

Educational Domain

There is little doubt that the women within physical education were timid in their approach to the Olympic competition. Perhaps the most accurate statement up until the 1960 Games would be that they were ambivalent about the 1948, 1952, and 1956 Games. DGWS's joining of the USOC through the multiple sports Class B membership in 1952 does, however, demonstrate some effort to be a part of the Olympic movement.[69] In the leadership of DGWS/NAGWS the policy statement changed more drastically as the new breed of leaders of the 1960s came into power. Katherine Ley, the most outspoken proponent of competitive athletics within the educational domain, commented:

> We must do two things: train the best we have to perform to the
> best of their ability, and at the same time promote all sports for
> all girls and women so that eventually we will have more prospects
> for the Olympics from which to choose the best.[70]

By 1960 the stage was set for the sport revolution for girls and women, since amateur and educational factions were now united in a loud, clear voice in support of the elite competitive experience. The AAU sought DGWS to

"Expand, improve, and coordinate programs involving Olympic activities in an effort to enrich women's Olympic ventures."[71] This effort bore fruit in 1963. The DGWS and the Women's Advisory Board of the Olympic Development Committee co-sponsored a series of five institutes for improvement of teaching and coaching in many of the Olympic and Pan-American sports. The first institute was held in 1963 in track and field and gymnastics. More than 200 teachers were instructed in teaching techniques for women's track and field and gymnastics, with the ensuing spin-off institutes resulting in more than 25,000 teachers and coaches being exposed to new approaches to training and coaching elite female athletes in track and field. This co-sponsorship was meaningful to both groups, not only for the expertise they gained and the ensuing "spin-off" institutes, but also because they helped to heal the wounds between the Olympic movement and physical educators.[72]

The new alliance between physical educators and the Olympic movement was aided by the most significant piece of legislation for sport in education, Title IX, which decreed that educational institutions may not discriminate on the basis of sex. This landmark legislation required varsity programs for girls if they were provided for boys. Opportunity was thus assured in sports for a whole generation of varsity-trained athletes, particularly in large popular sports like track and field and cross-country where there was a demonstrable desire to field a team but high schools and colleges had been reluctant to do so.

It was Title IX, of course, that mandated athletic scholarships for women and thus for the first time in history provided an opportunity for a combination of an education and athletic training for the world-class female athlete. It is clear that the women's Olympic track teams since 1976 have been made up of larger numbers of women who have gone through collegiate programs before their Olympic experience. These include distance runners like Doris Brown and Mary Decker, the marathon runner Joan Benoit, and sprinter Evelyn Ashford. The 1984 Olympic athletes reaped the harvest of the growth in intercollegiate athletic programs.

The NAGWS and its substructure, the Association for Intercollegiate Athletics for Women (AIAW) was the governing body for intercollegiate athletics from 1971 until its demise in 1982, when the control of intercollegiate athletics for women moved to the National Collegiate Athletic Association (NCAA). It was within the AIAW that state, regional, and national championships were conducted throughout the country. In its last full year of operation, 1980 to 1981, more than 99,000 female athletes participated in intercollegiate athletics under AIAW. In that year, AIAW held 39 championships in 17 sports, with more than 6,000 women's teams competing. In addition, there were 750 state, regional, and national preliminary tournaments. For example, in track and field, there were 532 institutions and in cross country, 440 institutions who fielded teams. Two hundred sixty-five institutions awarded financial aid based on track ability, and 199 did so for cross-country athletes, for a total spending of 4 million dollars for track and field athletes.[73] AIAW had a flexibility in its divisional structure that permitted sports like cross-country at a given institution to develop at their own pace, in keeping with the level of student interest, coaching expertise, funding, and popularity. This flexibility provided far greater opportunity for the development of new sport offerings in member institutions.

The success of Title IX has led to unbelievable growth in high school varsity teams for girls. Under the direction of state athletic associations, more than 1.8 million girls were on varsity teams in 1982 in 30 different sports. The High School Federation reports that in 1982 there were 397,000 athletes competing on more than 10,000 track-and-field teams.[74]

Besides expanding the number of varsity sport programs for girls and women and providing skilled sportswomen from all strata of society with the opportunity to attend college, Title IX had the less-apparent but nonetheless highly significant effect of improving the level of competition.

Popular Culture

Recreational centers were available for children and adults alike. Married women were able to pursue recreational sports either in female or mixed groups or with their spouses as part of the 1950s "togetherness" ethic. Their children (if male) took part in Little League baseball and football, or (if female) in some of the individual sports and cheerleading. Employers saw the value of having company teams and leagues, especially for the working woman. Communities, clubs, and churches also saw the value of sports for both the working woman and the home-bound mother.

AAU and Olympic Movement

A new era in Olympic competition began with the appearance of the USSR and Eastern bloc countries at the 1952 and 1956 Olympics. Their "instant gold medalists" reflected a higher degree of competitive intensity and training than previously evident. This forced the Western nations, including the United States, to seriously review their own programs. After the 1952 Games, manager-coach Lucile Wilson of the women's team commented on the well-organized track programs for boys in the school system and the lack of them for girls. She charged the educational institutions with depriving the girls and women of the chance to receive a proper and healthy program in track. Her words were echoed by Evelyne Hall, the chairman of the 1952 Track and Field Committee, who called women's track "the stepchild of American sports."[75] The news media noted the poor showing of the American female athletes in track and field and demanded more training. A New York reporter wrote (in nationalistic terms):

> If there was any lesson for us in the recent Olympics it may have been let's stop making track and field athletics a men's club only.

Let's strip away the chains which have kept women out of so many sports. For the Olympics were a warning: Women of other nations are getting ahead of us . . . it is we who are failing our girl athletes. . . . The eyes of the world are going to be on U.S. women in the 1956 Olympics.[76]

Roxanne Anderson, the 1956 coach, adds her concern: "The American girl is still fighting the Battle of Mid-Victorian prejudice against participation by women in competitive sport."[77] The educational establishment's failure to support rigorous competition was taking its toll.

Through television the 1960 Rome Olympics brought the true drama and glamour of competitive track and field, particularly the stellar performance of Wilma Rudolph, into homes, schools, and colleges throughout the world. Seeing Rudolph and the other world-class athletes amid the pageantry of the Games dispelled the idea that superb performances are achieved by "mesomorphic women with massive musculature." *Sports Illustrated*, and even Helen Gurley Brown in her popular *Sex and the Single Girl*, commented favorably on the value of track.[78]

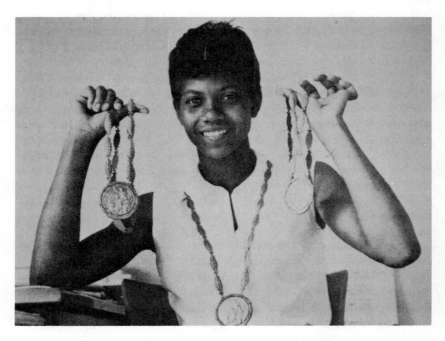

Figure 7   "Wilma Rudolph—Olympic Winner" (UPI photo). *Note.* From *100 Greatest Women in Sport,* by Phyllis Hollander, 1976, New York: Grosset and Dunlap. Reprinted with permission.

The success of track in the Olympics along with the new emphasis by the DGWS and Olympic development committee rekindled an interest in developing elite track athletes. The AAU expanded its track program and encouraged high schools and colleges to offer varsity teams; yet it lacked the necessary resources for a full-scale grass roots program. Without the necessary funding, had it not been for Tuskegee Institute and the Tennessee State University under the leadership of Edward Temple, American track records between 1948 and 1964 would have been even more dismal. At the height of their power in 1975, the AAU claimed more than 122,000 registered female athletes, with approximately 18,750 in track and field and 720 in long-distance running.[79]

A directional change in the purpose and structure of the AAU occurred in the mid 1970s for several reasons. First, there was the greater efficiency of The Athletic Congress of the United States (TAC), a new National Sport Governing Body (NGB), in a sort of "cradle to grave" servicing of an athlete in the sport. Second was a desire for unified male-female governance. Finally was the wish to resolve the destructive rivalry between the two athletic monoliths (the AAU and NCAA). One result of this directional change was that the TAC became the NGB of men's and women's track and field.[80]

A President's Commission on Olympic Sports 1975 to 1977 examined the entire Olympic structure, resulting in the Amateur Sports Act of 1978. The Act provided for 16 million dollars to restructure the entire Olympic movement and its NGB. Significant features of the new Act for long-distance runners were: (a) the development of a national headquarters for NGB and a training center for all Olympic sport teams in Colorado Springs, (b) a national sport festival each summer, (c) NGBs in all Olympic sports (AAU became TAC), (d) track and field and long-distance running for women were identified as "underdeveloped" sports (an underdeveloped sport demands that more funds be provided for grass root programs, training of elite athletes, and more research), (e) a Bill of Rights for the athletes. The Act is in itself responsible for revitalizing the Olympic program, bringing it on a par with those in the Eastern bloc countries, while attempting to maintain the United States ideal of nonprofessionalism.[81]

Summary

From 1950 through the mid 1980s, sport became much like American society itself in its heterogeneity and capacity for individuals to participate in diverse sports at different levels once the organized sport structure was in place. The previously divided stream of female athletics became a mighty river that finally enjoyed equal contributions and support from the educational domain and popular culture. For the first time there existed the unified network of the high school athletic associations, collegiate governances, and national sport governing bodies to act as a feeder system for the world-class athlete. With the advent of media coverage, which kindled the imagination and awareness of girls and women to their own potential, the promotion and availability of sport across the land, and infusion of federal legislation, the opportunities for girls and women in sport appeared limitless. Psychological and sociological patterns traced elsewhere in this volume also indicate that the American female now approaches athletics with a new self-confidence and pride.

Marathon

The struggle of the female marathoner for the opportunity to demonstrate her endurance and swiftness has been a long tedious route, almost as grueling as the event itself. The evidence is clear that the road to the Olympics for the marathoners and the 3,000-meter runners was not smooth, as has been the case with each new sport or event added to the Olympic program.

The marathon story may have started with a lone woman, Melpomene, but it ends with thousands of women on the road to Joan Benoit's victory. Between Melpomene's and Benoit's marathons, however, French, Mexican, South African, and British women all competed in men's marathons before the American Arlene Pieper's 1959 Marathon run up and down the Pike's Peak route. A less-publicized North American Hemisphere men's marathon run in Culver City, California, in 1963 featured two American females; one of the athletes, Merry Lepper, jumped in and finished the event in 3:37. The same year an unofficially recognized time of 3:27 was established by a Scotswoman, Dale Greig, who competed in the men's Isle of Wight Marathon.[82]

Perhaps the first milestone in the attack on the view of the popular culture and the top leadership of the male-dominated distance running occurred before the races of the early 1960s. This was the establishment in 1957 of the Road Runners Club of America (RRCA), which was the first organization that vowed to give women equal recognition.

In 1966 a 23-year-old California woman, Roberta Gibb, traveled across the country by bus to fulfill her dream of running in the Boston Marathon; unsure whether or not she would be barred from the race. Finding she could not officially enter, she jumped into the race and successfully completed the Boston route in 3:21. She was barely recognized for the achievement, either that year or the following year, when she again completed the run in 3:27 (well ahead of the more publicized Katherine Switzer's time).[83] Switzer officially entered the 1967 Boston Marathon by signing in as K.V. Switzer, and getting an official number. She was harrassed along the route by the race director; nonetheless, she unrelentingly finished the race in 4:20. Such were the new breed of distance runners who would be the role models for the female runners of the 1970s.[84]

The next decade and a half were indeed exciting and frustrating ones for the female long-distance runners. The freedom of running was experienced by thousands of women in hundreds of marathons. The event seems the perfect expression of the modern American temperament and time. Its popularity is, in part, an outgrowth of the national jogging movement that began in the mid 1970s with participants of both sexes. It reflects an increased interest in better health and improved self-image, and it is available at the nearest footpath. Even with an increase in the number of recreational runners from 1 million in 1975 to 19 million in 1985, the struggle for recognition for elite female runners was not an easy task.[85]

The first American National Women's Marathon Championship in October 1970 sponsored by the RRCA was the beginning of the organized marathon runs. By 1972, women had officially entered the Boston and New York Marathons. The first AAU championship for women occurred in 1974 (with men, and not as a separate event until 1977). The first Avon International Marathon was in 1978. During the 1970s the number of marathons increased. At almost all of the major races, the time barriers were lowered until by the end of the decade, the time of 2:27 had cut over one hour from the first 1963 unofficial time. The 1984 record stands at 2:22:43.[86]

In the struggle for entry into the Olympics, several important influences stand out. The greatest boost to American marathon running was provided by the entrance of Avon Products into elite and grass roots running programs, not only in the United States, but in foreign countries as well. They not only sponsored the events but even paid all expenses to ensure that the top marathon runners could attend. Dr. Ernest Van Aaken held two international marathons in his home town of Waldniel, West Germany (1974 & 1976) before the first Avon sponsored marathon, absorbing most of the expenses. These actions satisfied the Olympic requirement that a sport should be "practiced widely in 25 countries and on two continents." Both Dr. Van Aaken's 1979 and Avon's 1980 Marathons fulfilled this requirement. The tremendous success of the marathons had given visibility to female athletes everywhere except in the governance structures of the Olympic movement.[87]

The first battle for recognition by the AAU continued until 1972 when they finally rescinded the 10-mile limit for female runners. Next was the IAAF meeting in Montreal in 1976, when the USOC-backed request for the 3,000-meter and marathon races were both denied with only brief discussion. As a result of this loss, the marathoners themselves gathered volunteers, compiled research data, and politically moved toward a victory for the 1984 Olympics. In keeping with this goal, the International Runners' Committee (IRC) was founded to lobby for the inclusion of distance runners in the Olympics. Key personnel in this effort included Jacqueline Hansen, Joe Henderson, Lealann Reinhart, and Nina Kuscsik (who chairs TAC's Women's Long Distance Committee).[88]

The year 1979 ended with the Women's International Marathon being held in downtown Tokyo, featuring world-class runners. The president of IAAF, Adrian Paulsen, attended the event and was so impressed that he became an active campaigner for the marathon for the Women's 1984 Olympics by writing extensively about the event, praising the women runners, and encouraging immediate action for the 3,000-meter run and the marathon. He comments in an IRC newsletter:

> The athletes running today, by careful preparation and gradual buildup, are, therefore, ready for the challenge which the summit of distance races presents. . . . the great impetus of women's long distance running continues, and the movement will gather more and more support.[89]

And so it did, with financial backing from Nike, and with volunteers through the IRC working from every angle to encourage the leaders of the IAAF and the IOC in Moscow to accept the petition for the 1984 marathon. The petition was defeated, however, as the leadership asked for more evidence regarding physiological factors. More medicoscientific data was collected and provided for the next battle.

Several victories at the 1980 Moscow meeting, however, were:

1. The 1980 IAAF ruled that all international events with men's marathons would also have races for women,
2. The IAAF recognized the 5,000 and 10,000 as official world-record distances,
3. The 3,000-meter race would be in the 1984 Olympics, and
4. The decision on the marathon for the 1984 Olympic Games would be postponed until the 1981 meeting.

At the meeting early in 1981, the IOC refused to sanction the marathon for women. It would take an additional campaign by the IRC and other running enthusiasts to reverse that decision through the intervention of the IAAF and later through the support of the Los Angeles Olympic Organizing Committee. (Originally, the LAOOC protested the addition of the event.)[90]

In a careful analysis of the political situation and the difficulties encountered in getting the marathon on the Olympic program, Jacqueline Hansen, herself a world-record holder in the marathon, a long-distance runner, and one of the founders of the IRC, commented

> The IOC appears to have felt terribly threatened by the women's running movement. Perhaps beneath all of the organization's [IOC's] physiological and political arguments lay the cultural and psychological problems that, while less common today, have plagued the athletic establishment.[91]

On February 23, 1981, the Executive Committee of the IOC met to reconsider the marathon question. Several IRC members and interested marathoners were present to campaign.[92] Finally, after almost four generations of women had missed an opportunity to compete for the gold in the Olympics, the Women's Marathon would be added to the roster of the 1984 Olympic Events.

Conclusion

Melpomene was the first "invisible" female runner, invisible because although she ran the marathon in 1896, no record suggests her presence. She was a nonperson to the power structure, which at that time saw the full expanse of the human condition borne only in its own male image. American women were invisible politically until federal legislation accorded them their political rights. Women were invisible in the mirror as long as they were a reflection of their own socialization process. In 1981 female marathoners were all invisible to the Olympic leadership that decided women were not able to run the marathon, despite the fact that they were already doing it.

Seen over the past century, 1880 to the present, the elite female athlete's quest for visibility is very like the marathon itself, with generations of elite athletes learning along the torturous route the value of:

- identity and selfhood;
- political tenacity in fighting discrimination and gaining rights;
- the necessity for engaging in a power struggle where necessary and surrendering comfortable academic isolation;
- role models who have boldly stepped outside the sex role expectations of their peers;
- motivation in the face of cultural disapproval resulting from the socialization process;
- sport programs and leadership development;
- training and mentorship; and
- a unique female sport tradition.

It took centuries of struggle for Benoit to cross the Olympic finish line, and in fact the thousands of distance runners today attest to present visibility and potential of the world class female athlete. Benoit, because of the preeminence women's sport has now achieved, is not seen as an anomaly or "a credit to her sex." Her struggle was not just female, it was human, as writer Candace Lyle Hogan suggests:

> Sportswomen had become suddenly, obviously overqualified for the role of "symbol of the capable female;" experiencing the worst and best of days right before our eyes, they were clearly made of profoundly universal stuff. In their joys, their desire and their misfortune, they mirrored the human condition to us.[93]

Equally poignant and memorable to the millions who watched the Olympic Marathon on television in 1984 was the sight of Switzerland's Gabriele Andersen-Schiess, near delirious from heat exhaustion, painfully zig-zagging

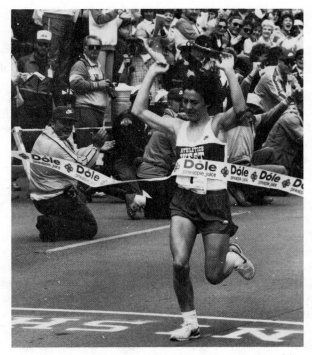

Figure 8   Joan Benoit crosses the finish line. Photo courtesy of the
Weyerhaeuser Company.

her way around the last lap to the tape. A commentator covering the event
said that he could see her condition even before she entered the Los Angeles
Coliseum and was in a dilemma as to whether to report her situation. Should
the world see the picture worth a thousand words that might endanger the future
of distance running for women?

But there was no repeat of the 1928 Olympic disaster because the views
of physical educators and the popular culture have changed over time regarding the worth and potential of the female athlete. The marathon, therefore,
is in no danger of being lost to the Olympics. The female American runner
has won her modern quest for visibility, and the freedom to strive for the
Olympic gold. And somewhere below that state of delirium experienced by
Andersen-Schiess is the heightened mystical experience found in the act of
competitive distance running. This psychic and reflective path to self-knowledge
is in the nature of the marathon experience whereby the elite athlete has been
freed to discover so keenly both the agony and the ecstasy of being human.

Notes

1. Simri, U. (1977). *A historical analysis of the role of women in the modern Olympic games* (p. 6). Nitanya, Israel: Wingate Institute of Physical Education and Sport.

2. Foldes, E. (1964). Women at the Olympics. *The International Olympic Academy, Report of the Fourth Session* (p. 108). Athens: Pechlivandis, as cited in Welch, P. (1975). *The emergence of American women in the summer Olympic games: 1900-1972* (pp. 11-12). Doctoral dissertation, University of North Carolina at Greensboro.

3. Eisen, G. (1975). *Sports and women in antiquety* (pp. 244, 251, 263-264). Master's thesis, University of Massachusetts. *See also* Gardiner, E.N. (1970). *Greek athletics, sports and festivals* (pp. 47, 49, 239, 462). Dubuque, IA: Wm. C. Brown Reprints.

4. Orwell, G. (1968). Marrakech. In C. Muscatine & M. Griffith (Eds.), *The Borzoi College reader* (p. 269). New York: Knopf.

5. Gardiner, *Greek athletics, sports and festivals*, pp. 40-41, 46-49, 239, 386-387, 462. See also Robinson, R.S. (1955). *Sources for the history of Greek athletics* (p. 109-163). Cincinnati, OH: Author. See also Harris, H.A., (1972). *Sport in Greece and Rome*, (pp. 40-41, 64-65). Ithaca, NY: Cornell University Press.

6. Harris, H.A. (1964). *Greek athletes and athletics* (pp. 179-186). London: Hutchinson. *See also* Balsdon, U.P.V.D. (1969). *Life and leisure in ancient Rome* (pp. 67-168, 290-291, 297-299). New York: McGraw-Hill.

7. Eisen, *Sports and women in antiquety,* pp. 100-102, 254-55, 263.

8. Eisen, *Sports and women in antiquety,* pp. 214-244; Gardiner, *Greek athletics, sports, and festivals,* pp. 47, 239, 462; Robinson, 109-163, 266.

9. Harris, *Greek athletes and athletics,* pp. 40-41.

10. LaRousse, P.G. (1965). *World mythology* (p. 152). London: Hamlyn.

11. Tyler, M.C. (1967). *A history of American literature, 1607-1783* (pp. 85-86). Chicago: Phoenix Books, University of Chicago Press.

12. Hints on riding. (1878, July). *Godey's Lady's Book and Magazine*, Vol. 97, pp. 70-71. *See also* The sailing race at the spring meet of the Hudson River Canoe Club. (1885, June 13). *Harper's Weekly*, p. 376. *See also* Skating for ladies. (1863, December). *Godey's Lady's Magazine*, Vol. 67, pp. 567-568. *See also* Swimming. (1858, August). *Godey's Lady's Magazine*, Vol. 57, pp. 123-125.

13. Beecher, C. (1855) *Letters to the people on health and happiness* (pp. 168-171). New York: Harper & Brothers, as cited in Lockhart, A.S., and Spears, B. (1972). *Chronicle of American physical education* (pp. 3-9). Dubuque, IA: Brown. *See also* Midwest Association of College Teachers of Physical Education for Women. (1951). *A century of growth: The historical development of physical education for women in selected colleges of six midwestern states*. Ann Arbor, MI: Edwards Brothers. *See also* Richardson, S.F.

(1897, February). Tendencies in athletics for women in colleges and universities. *Popular Science*, Vol. 50, pp, 517-526. *See also* Shaw, A. (1892, December). Physical culture at Wellesley. *Review of Reviews*, Vol. 6, pp. 545-547.

14. Benough, B. (1896, January). The new woman athletically considered. *Godey's Lady's Magazine*, Vol. 132, pp. 23-29. *See also* Ayres, W. (1895, July). Smith College. *Godey's Lady's Magazine*, Vol. 131, p. 25.

15. Remley, M.L. (1984, May) *The steel-engraving lady and the Gibson girl: The American sportswoman in transition: 1880-1910* (pp. 3-7). Paper presented at the 12th Annual Convention of the North American Society for Sport History, University of Louisville. *See also* Wells, K.G. (1880, December). The transitional American woman. *Atlantic Monthly*, p. 819. *See also* Cumming, J. *Runners and walkers: A nineteenth century sports chronicle* (pp. 102-104). Chicago: Regnery Gateway.

16. Cumming, *Runners and walkers* . . . , 102.

17. Cumming, *Runners and walkers* . . . , 103-104.

18. Cavallo D. (1981). *Muscles and morals: Organized playgrounds and urban reform, 1880-1920* (pp. 32-48, 55-65, 110-124). Philadelphia: University of Pennsylvania Press. *See also* Lucas, J.A., and Smith, R.A. (1978). *Saga of American sport* (pp. 287-301. Philadelphia, Lea & Febiger.

19. Cavallo, *Muscles and morals* . . . , pp. 110-124.

20. Spears, B. The emergence of women in sport. In B.J. Hoepner (Ed.), *Women's athletics: Coping with controversy* (pp. 26-39). Washington, D.C.: American Association for Health, Physical Education, and Recreation. *See also* Hult, J.S. (1985). The governance of athletic for girls and women: Leadership by women physical educators, 1899-1949. *Research Quarterly in Exercise and Sport*, Centennial Issue, pp. 91-115. *See also* Ballintine, H. (1898, March). Out-of-door sports for college women. *American Physical Education Review*, **3**, 38-43.

21. Wells, The transitional American woman, p. 819.

22. Matthaei, J. (1982). *An economic history of women in America: Women's work, the sexual division of labor, and the development of capitalism* (pp. 203-205, 209-213). New York: Schocken. *See also* Woody, T. (1929). *A history of women's education in the U.S. II* (pp. 639-649). New York: Science Press. *See also* Crusade against the wheel for women. (1896, July). *The Literary Digest*, Vol. 13, p. 361. *See also* Herrick, T.H. (1902, September). Women in athletics: The athletic girl not unfeminine. *Outing*, Vol. 26, pp. 712-721.

23. Dickinson, R.L. (1896, April 25). Bicycling for women: The puzzling question of costume. *Outlook*, pp. 751-752. *See also* Merington, M. (1897). Women and the bicycle. *Athletic Sports—The Out-of-Door Library*, Vol. 5, pp. 209-230. *See also* Dress reform in Boston. (1874). *Herald of Health and Journal of Physical Culture*, Vol. 58, pp. 71-73.

24. Willard, F.E. (1895). *A wheel within a wheel*. Chicago: Woman's Temperance Publishing Association.

25. LeLong, M.V. (1898, February & March). From Chicago to San Francisco Awheel. *Outing*, Vol. 22, pp. 492-497, 592-596.

26. Kerber, L.K., & Mathews, J.D. (Eds.). (1982). *Women's America: Refocusing the past* (pp. 257-260). New York: Oxford University Press. *See also* Frankfort, R. (1977). *Collegiate women* (p. 87). New York: New York University Press.

27. Pinkham, L.E. (undated). *Lydie E. Pinkham's private textbook upon ailments peculiar to women* (p. 21). Lynn, MA: Pinkham Medicine Co.

28. Berenson, S. (1901). Editorial in *Basket ball for women, 1901* (pp. 5-7). New York: American Sports.

29. Hult, J.S. (1980). *Have the reports of the death of competitive women's athletics 1920-35 been greatly exaggerated?* Paper presented at the Seventh Annual Convention of the North American Society for Sport History, Banff, Canada. *See also* Stewart, H. (1916, January). A survey of track athletics for women. *American Physical Education Review,* **21,** 13-21.

30. Amateur Athletic Union of the United States. (1914, November). *Minutes of Annual Meeting, November 1914* (p. 25). New York. *See also* idem. (1916, November). *Minutes of Annual Meeting, November 1916.* New York.

31. Stewart, H. (1914, February). The effect on the heart rate and blood pressure of vigorous athletics in girls. *American Physical Education Review,* **19,** 119. *See also* idem. A survey of track, pp. 13-21.

32. Peiss, K. (1984, May). *The exploitation of pleasure: The commercialization of working-class women's leisure, 1880-1920.* Paper presented at the Leisure-Time Business Conference, Wilmington, DE. *See also* Gulick, L. The social function of play (Gulick Papers, Springfield College, MA) as cited in Cavallo, *Muscles and morals . . . ,* pp. 125-146. *See also* New York American Sports Publishing Co. (1901-1930). *The Women's Sport Guide in Basketball and Track and Field.*

33. $5,000 in prizes to physical culture enthusiasts. (1903, November). *Beauty and Health,* pp. 332-333, as quoted in Remley, *The steel-engraving lady.*

34. Mitchell, S. (1977, Summer). Women's participation in the Olympic games: 1900-1926. *Journal of Sport History,* **4,** 214.

35. Amateur Athletic Union of the United States. (1914, November). *Minutes of Annual Meeting, November 1914* (p. 25). New York. *See also* idem, (1916, November). *Minutes of Annual Meeting, November 1916* (p. 31). New York. *See also* Dawson, B. (Ed.). (1971). Hall of fame pick for mythical U.S. Olympic swimming teams. *International Swimming Hall of Fame, fifth anniversary yearbook: 1965-1970* (pp. 136-137). Fort Lauderdale, FL: International Swimming Hall of Fame.

36. Hult, *Have the reports of the death of competitive women's athletics 1920-35 been greatly exaggerated?*

37. Davidson, J.A. (1978). *The 1930's: A pivotal decade for women's sport.* Unpublished qualifying manuscript, University of Massachusetts.

38. Gerber, E.W. (1975, Spring). The controlled development of collegiate sport for women, 1923-1936. *Journal of Sport History, 2,* 1-28. *See also* Hult, *Have the reports of the death of competitive women's athletics 1920-35 been greatly exaggerated?* and Hult, The governance of athletics for girls and women, pp. 100-106.

39. Federal Security Agency, U.S. Office of Education (1943). *Physical fitness for students in college and universities,* (pp. 50-59, 83) and *Physical fitness through education for the Victory Corps.* Washington, D.C.: Government Printing Office.

40. American Physical Education Association. (1922, September). Report of the business meeting, May, 1922. *American Physical Education Review, 27,* 332-335.

41. Burchenal, E. (1923). *Official handbook of the National Committee on Women's Athletics and the official rules for swimming, track and field, and soccer, 1923-1924.* New York: American Sports. For a history of the Women's Division, see Sefton, A.A. (1941). *The Women's Division National Amateur Athletic Federation.* Stanford, CA: Stanford University Press. For a history of CWA/NSWA/DGWS, see Hult, J.S., *The governance of athletics,* pp. 91-100.

42. Wayman, A. (1938). *A modern philosophy of physical education* (p. 170). Philadelphia: Saunders.

43. Burchenal, *Official handbook . . . ,* pp. 1-14. *See also* Trilling, B. (1929, August). The playtime of a million girls or an Olympic victory: Which? *The Nation's Schools,* Vol. 6, p. 52. *See also* Women's Division National Amateur Athletic Federation. (1924). *WDNAAF Platform.* New York: WDNAAF. *See also* Perrin, E. (1929, February). More competitive athletics for girls—but of the right kind. *American Physical Education Review, 34,* 473-476.

44. Bell, M. (1938). *The doctor answers some practical questions on menstruation.* Washington, D.C.: American Association for Health, Physical Education, And Recreation (AAHPER). *See also* National Section on Women's Athletics. (1941). *Desirable practices for girls and women in sport.* New York: Barnes.

45. Wayman, A. (1924, November). Women's athletics: All uses—no abuses. *American Physical Education Review, 29,* 517.

46. Burchenal, *Official handbook . . . ,* pp. 14-15. *See also* National Section on Women's Athletics (1937). *Standards in athletics for girls and women.* Washington, D.C.: AAHPER. *See also* Hult, *The governance of athletics,* pp. 104-106.

47. Gittings, I. (1931). Why camp competition? *Journal of Health and Physical Education, 2,* 10.

48. Hult, *Have the reports of the death of competitive women's athletics . . . ? See also* Coops, H. (1926, November). Sports for American women. *American Physical Education Review, 31,* 1086. *Also* Women's Division

National Amateur Athletic Federation. Unpublished special reports from recreational and industrial centers from 1925-1928 to 1929-1930 in Women's Division AAHPERD Archives. *See also* Hiss, A. (1937, February). Basketball leagues: What about them and our responsibilities? *Journal of Health and Physical Education*, **8**, 104.

49. Hult, *Have the reports of the death of competitive women's athletics . . . ? See also* Borries, E. Questionnaire results compiled in recreational and industrial files of Women's Division of AAHPERD Archives. *See also Official rules of women's basketball, 1924-25 & 1925-1926.* New York: American Sports. *See also* Gates, E., (1929, June). Trends in athletics for girls and women in employed groups. *American Physical Education Review*, **34**, 366.

50. Hult, J. (1982, April). *The role of women physical educators and organizations in American women's struggle for the Olympic gold: 1922-1968.* Paper presented at the 97th Annual Convention of AAHPERD, Houston. *See also* National Section on Women's Athletics. (1929, May). News of girls and women's athletics. *American Physical Education Review*, **34**, 310. *See also* Wayman, A. (1932, March). Women's Division of the National Amateur Athletic Federation. *Journal of Health and Physical Education*, **3**, 45. *See also* National Section on Women's Athletics. (1935, April). *Minutes of the Legislative Board of NSWA.*

51. Becker, O. (1934, February). Ex-Champion Now Chairman. *Amateur Athlete*, pp. 11-12. *See also* American Physical Education Association Council. (1934). Basketball Committee Report. *See also* Vinson, M.Y. (1936, July 12). Women in sports. *The New York Times,* sec. V., p. 6.

52. Woman's Sports Committee of the Amateur Athletic Union. (1933). *The Sportswoman*, **9**, 21. *See also* the NSWA Basketball Committee's undated report to the American Physical Education Association entitled, ''Request to rescind 1932 ruling.'' *See also* J. Griffith's letter of 1931, May 27, to E. Perrin concerning AAU/NSWA conflicts. *See also* NSWA. (1932, April 20-23). *Memorandum of activities of Women's Athletic Editorial Committee.*

53. Wohlford, M. (1947, January). NSWA national convention. *Sports Bulletin*, p. 10. *See also* NSWA. (1947, January). *Minutes of the Legislative Board Meeting. See also* Remley, M.L. (1970). *Twentieth-century concepts of sports competition for women.* (pp. 20-25, 32-38). Doctoral dissertation, University of Southern California. *See also* Schriver, A. (1949, September). Competition: NSWA faces the issue. *Journal of Health, Physical Education, and Recreation,* **20**, 472.

54. Hult, J.S., & Park, R. (1981). The role of women in sports. In W.J. Baker and J.M. Carroll (Eds.), *Sports in modern America* (pp. 115-128). St. Louis: River City.

55. Leigh, M.H. (1977, Spring). The pioneering role of Madame Alice Milliat and the FSFI in establishing international track and field competition for women. *Journal of Sport History,* **4**, 72-83.

56. Stewart, S. (1922, June). Track athletics for women. *American Physical Education Review, 27*, 288.

57. Steers, F.L. (1923). Report of Committee on Women's Athletics, November 1923; Report of Committee on Women's Athletics National Convention, New York, 1922. *Minutes of the Amateur Athletic Union (AAU) of the United States, 1923,* (p. 142). These reports may be found in the AAU Archives, Indianapolis.

58. Steers, F.L. Report of Committee on Women's Athletics, November 1923 (pp. 138-139) (AAU Archives).

59. Steers, F.L. (1925). Report of Committee on Women's Athletics, November 1924. *Minutes of the AAU, 1924* (pp. 73-76). *See also* Report of Committee on Women's Athletics, November 1925. *Minutes of the AAU, November 1925* (pp. 110-111) (AAU Archives).

60. Sayers, T. (1927, June). Track and field. *Athletic Journal, 3*, 20-24. *See also* Questionnaire results, 1923, *Official track and field athletics for girls, 1924* and Questionnaire results, 1924, *Official track and field athletics for girls, 1925.* New York: American Sports.

61. Welch, P. (1975). *The emergence of American women in the summer Olympic games: 1900-1972* (pp. 41-42). Doctoral dissertation, University of North Carolina at Greensboro. *See also* Webster, F.A.M. (1930). *Athletics of to-day for women: History, development and training* (p. 11). London: Warne.

62. Steers, F.L. (1927). Report of Committee on Women's Athletics, November 1927; Report of the Committee on Women's Athletics National Convention, Cincinnati, 1927. *Minutes of the Amateur Athletic Union, 1927* (AAU Archives).

63. Steers, F.L. (1928). Report of manager of women's track and field team. *Report of the American Olympic Committee.* New York: American Olympic Committee. *See also* Pallet, G. (1955). *Women's athletics* (pp. 37-50). London: Normal Press. *See also* Webster, *Athletics of to-day* (p. 110).

64. Tunis, J. (1929, July). Women and the sport business. *Harper's Monthly*, p. 213.

65. International Amateur Athletic Federation (IAAF). (1930). *Minutes of the 10th Congress of the IAAF, Berlin. See also* Kirby, G.T. (1929, March). The 1928 Olympics. *The Playground*, p. 718. *See also* Kirby boycotts the track men. (1930, May 21). *The New York Evening Post.*

66. Simri, *A historical analysis of the role of women . . . ,* p. 21.

67. Simri, *A historical analysis of the role of women . . . ,* p. 21-22.

68. Friedan, B. (1963). *The feminine mystique.* New York: Dell.

69. Remley, *Twentieth-century concepts of sports competition for women,* pp. 60-62, 79-81.

70. Ley, K. (1965). A philosophical interpretation of the National Institute on Girls' Sports. *Proceedings of the First National Institute on Girls' Sports* (p. 12). Washington, D.C.: AAHPER.

71. Jernigan, S.S. (1962, April). Women and the Olympics. *Journal of Health, Physical Education, and Recreation, 32*, 26.

72. Jernigan, Women and the Olympics, p. 25-26. *See also* Jernigan, S.S. (1984, March). Interview of DGWS women in the Olympic movement. Paper presented at the National AAHPERD Convention, Anaheim, CA. *See also* Jernigan, S.S. (1969). Foreword. *Proceedings of the Fifth National Institute on Girls' Sports.* Washington, D.C.: AAHPER. *See also* Stiles M.H. (1968). A new look at Olympic sports development. *Proceedings of the Fourth National Institute on Girls' Sports* (pp. 20-23). Washington, D.C.: AAHPER.

73. Uhlir, A. (1982, November). The wolf is our shepherd: Shall we not fear? *Phi Delta Kappan,* Vol. 64, p. 173. *See also Association of Intercollegiate Athletics for Women (AIAW) Sports Statistics by Division and Region, 1981-1982,* available in AIAW Archives, University of Maryland. *See also* Uhlir, A. (1984, Winter). For Whom Does the Money Toll? *Journal of the National Association of Women Deans, Administrators, and Counselors.*

74. National Federation of State High School Associations (NFSHSA). (1981). *Sports participants survey, 1971-1981,* available in NFSHSA files, Kansas City, MO.

75. Wilson, L. (1952). Women's track and field report of team manager-coach in A.S. Bushnell (Ed.), *United States 1952 Olympic Book* (p. 112). New Haven: Walker-Rackliff. *See also* Hall, E.R. (1952). Woman's track and field report of the Committee on women's athletics. In Bushnell, U.S. 1952 Olympic Book, p. 112.

76. Ferris, D.J. (1952, October). Let's have more coed sports. *The Amateur Athlete,* p. 17. Reprinted from *Parade Magazine.* 1952, September 28.

77. Welsh, *The emergence of women* . . . , p. 124.

78. Kaszubski, F. (undated). A rediscovery. *Olympic Sports* (p. 28). New York: U.S. Olympic Committee. *See also* Welsh, *The Emergence of Women* . . . , p. 141.

79. President's Commission on Olympic Sports. (1977). *Final Report.* (Vol. II). Washington, D.C.: Government Printing Office. *See also* Bentsen, C. (1978, February). Tigerbelle tradition. *Women's Sports,* Vol. 5, pp. 42-45, 52-53.

80. President's Commission on Olympic Sports. (1977). *Final Report,* Vols. I & II, pp. 221-234.

81. Amateur Sport Act of 1978; Report of the Senate Committee on Commerce, Science, and Transportation. Washington, D.C.: Government Printing Office. *See also* Ulrich, C. (1977, October-November). Soon it may be too late. (pp. 10-11).

82. Switzer, K.V. (1982, December). Running through history. *Women's Sports,* Vol. 4, pp. 27-28.

83. Hollander, P. (1976). *100 greatest women in sports* (pp. 139-140). New York: Grosset & Dunlap.

84. Hansen, J. (1984, September). Women's marathon movement: We've run a long way (Part One). *Marathon Newsletter,* p. 3. Seattle: Women's Marathon Trials Association.

85. Figures reported to the Women's Sport Foundation, San Francisco, CA, by the President's Council on Physical Fitness (1984, Fall). Also, Amdur, N. (1983, April 20). Women make big gains in marathon. *The New York Times* pp. B-12, B-17. *See also* Cimons, M. (1981, July). How women got to run the distance. *Ms* magazine, pp. 47-50.

86. Lewis, A.G. (1977, October-November). Women's national AAU marathon. *Sportswoman*, pp. 55-56. *See also* Hansen, J. (1984). Women's marathon movement: We've run a long way. (Part One, September; Part Two, October; Part Three, November). *Marathon Newsletter*. Seattle: Women's Marathon Trials Association. *See also* Hansen, J. (1984). Women make their own way. *Marathoning '84* (pp. 65-68). Mt. View, CA: Runner's World.

87. Hansen, Women's marathon movement. *See also* Hansen, Women make their own way. *See also* Switzer, K. (1983). Brief chronology of women's distance running (mimeograph). New York: Avon International Running Circuit.

88. Hansen, Women's marathon movement. *See also* Henderson, J. (1984, December). How the women's Olympic marathon was born. *Marathon Newsletter*, p. 10. Seattle: Women's Marathon Trials Association.

89. Paulsen, A. *International Runners' Committee Newsletter* as cited in Hansen, Women's marathon movement, Part Three.

90. Hansen, Women's marathon movement. *See also* Hansen, Women make their own way. *See also* Henderson, J. (1985, January). How the women's Olympic marathon was born (Part Two). *Marathon Newsletter*.

91. Hansen, Women's marathon movement, Part Three.

92. Cimons, How women run got to run . . . *See also* Hansen, Women's marathon movement. *See also* Henderson, How the women's Olympic marathon was born.

93. Hogan, C.L. (1984, October). An Olympic inspiration. *The Runner,* Vol. 7, p. 32.

2 Women and Endurance: Some Factors Influencing Performance

Jacqueline L. Puhl

Sports Medicine Division
United States Olympic Committee

Over the centuries sport has been a mirror of society—a reflection of sociocultural attitudes, beliefs, and phenomena. Until the last 10 to 15 years, the limited participation of women in sport, particularly endurance activities, reflected society's view that women were capable of many physical stresses associated with everyday living but were not considered able to participate in endurance sports and activities associated with leisure pursuits. During the past decade, the ramifications of increasing interest in health and fitness and of Title IX have become apparent. Now women of all ages are not only active in almost all phases of the work force, they are also participating in all types of sports, physical activities, and exercise programs. The boom in women's participation in sport and exercise and the parallel increase in the number of well-trained women has given impetus to research on physiological differences and similarities between men and women at all levels of fitness and stages of training. Today's woman is more active than before and today's woman athlete is training as hard as her male counterpart. Consequently, physiological and performance differences that existed a decade ago may be diminished or no longer exist.

Many factors can influence women's performance in endurance activities. Those physiological factors chosen for review are body composition, muscle characteristics, and energy supply. At the outset of this review, there are several basic concepts to be recognized. Some biological sex differences may affect sport performance. However, there is considerable overlap between men and women not only in performance but in physiological characteristics that may influence performance. When gender differences are observed, actual biological differences and the effects of training should be differentiated. Although there may be gender differences in the magnitude of response of a particular physiological characteristic to training, the relative amount and rate of adaptation appear to be similar when training stress is relative and the initial fitness levels are the same. Finally, there are questions yet to be answered. These answers and the insight they provide may have implications for women and their training programs.

Body Size and Composition

In addition to obvious sex differences in height and weight, men and women also differ in body composition. The average man has a larger proportion of muscle and a lower percentage of body fat than the average woman. The result of these differences is that men possess a greater lean body weight (muscle, bone, and organs) and a larger total muscle mass. Height and weight may be important in some, but not all, sports. However, a larger amount and/or proportion of muscle is usually an advantage in most sports.

In general, women have about 8% to 10% more body fat than men (Sparling, 1980). Reported values of percent body fat vary from about 13% to 16% fat and 22% to 26% fat for young adult men and women, respectively (Sparling, 1980). Many athletic groups, both male and female, have a lower percentage of body fat than their sedentary peers (Drinkwater, 1984; Fleck, 1983; Sparling, 1980; Wilmore, 1974; Wilmore, 1979). Athletes are often taller and heavier than the average person and frequently heavier than individuals their same height. This body weight difference reflects a larger total muscle mass common to many athletes (Fleck, 1983). The gender difference in percent body fat is usually less between male and female athletes of the same sport than in the general population (Fleck, 1983; Haymes & Dickenson, 1980; Puhl, Case, Fleck, & Van Handel, 1982; Sinning, Cunningham, Racaniello, & Sholes, 1977; Sparling, 1980; Wilmore, 1976). In elite endurance athletes, the gender difference in percent body fat is often rather small (2% to 6%) (Wilmore, 1976). Although there are biological reasons (higher estrogen and lower testosterone levels) for the higher percentage of body fat and lower percentage of muscle in women, less difference between men and women in the same sport suggests that part of the gender difference may be related to training and/or a reflection of sociocultural influence on participation.

As a factor influencing performance, body composition is more important in some sports than in others. Body composition may have relatively little influence on performance in some low-energy-cost sports (for example, archery and golf), although muscle mass and strength may be important. Aesthetics and appearance can be aspects of performance (and score) influenced by body composition in sports such as diving, synchronized swimming, gymnastics, and rhythmic gymnastics. Muscle mass affects strength, power, muscular endurance, and speed, which in turn influence many types of sport performance. Because of their typically higher percentage of body fat and lower total muscle mass, women are often at a disadvantage in sports where force and power are essential. Additionally, body fat does not contribute to movement and, in fact, is an extra load that can hinder performance in weight-bearing and loco-motor activities. Thus, body composition is important in sports where the athlete must move his/her body weight and in sports where athletes compete by weight class.

Muscle Characteristics

Skeletal muscles provide the force for body movements and stability for other body parts during movements. In sport, we observe the effectiveness of muscle function in performance. How a muscle functions in producing a movement is influenced by the types of muscle fibers it contains, their innate as well as training-enhanced metabolic capabilities, and the control of various fibers within the muscle and between the various muscles involved.

Muscle Fiber Types and Characteristics

Human skeletal muscles are composed of long, thin cells called fibers. There are different types of muscle fibers within a single skeletal muscle. Skeletal muscle fibers are grouped into motor units (functional contractile units) in which all fibers within a given motor unit are homogenous (consist of one fiber type) (Garnett, O'Donovan, Stephens, & Taylor, 1978; Saltin & Gollnick, 1984). The fibers in a motor unit are usually interspersed throughout the muscle resulting in a mosaic pattern of different fiber types.

Skeletal muscle fibers have been described based on their contractile and metabolic characteristics (Gans, 1982; Gollnick & Sembrowich, 1977; Saltin, Henriksson, Nygaard, Jansson, & Anderson, 1977; Saltin & Gollnick, 1984). Based on their contractile characteristics, they are classified as slow twitch (ST) and fast twitch (FT). Histochemical evidence indicates that in several mammalian species, there are subgroups of both fast (Type II) and slow twitch (Type I) fibers (Gollnick, Parsons, & Oakley, 1983; Saltin et al., 1977; Saltin & Gollnick, 1984). Both speed of contraction (time to peak isometric tension) and maximal contractile force differ between fiber types. As the fiber type names describe, FT fibers reach their peak isometric tension more rapidly than ST fibers (Saltin & Gollnick, 1984). In addition to having a faster contraction rate, FT fibers also reach higher peak tensions than ST fibers, although some contradictory evidence exists. Saltin and Gollnick (1984) concluded that in humans, the capacity of ST fibers to develop force per cross-sectional area does not appear to be significantly different from that of FT fibers. Additional research and more sophisticated techniques may provide insight into the similar-ities and differences in contractile properties of muscle fiber types.

The metabolic properties (substrate concentrations and enzyme activities) of the muscle fiber types support their contractile characteristics. ST fibers have a relatively high capacity for aerobic metabolism, whereas FT fibers generally have a higher capacity for anaerobic metabolism. However, subgroups of FT fibers appear to portray differences in aerobic/anaerobic potentials (Saltin et al., 1977; Saltin & Gollnick, 1984). The different types also vary in their fatigue characteristics (i.e. some fibers fatigue more rapidly than others). In general, FT fibers fatigue more rapidly than ST fibers. However, FT subgroups apparently have a spectrum of fatigue characteristics ranging from fast-fatiguing fibers to fatigue-resistant fibers (Garnett et al., 1978; Saltin & Gollnick, 1984). The implications of these force, metabolic, and fatigue characteristics for performance are that ST fibers are well suited for submaximal force production associated with prolonged endurance exercise, and FT fibers are generally better suited for larger force production associated with short-term, high-intensity exercise, although some FT fibers have greater endurance capabilities than others.

The muscle fiber recruitment pattern during physical activities reflects the characteristics of the muscle fiber types. Recruitment of muscle fibers (motor units) during physical activity depends on the intensity of the exercise (Gollnick & Sembrowich, 1977) and, in nonfatigued muscle, the tension or force needed for the task. The greater the exercise intensity or force required, the more muscle fibers (motor units) recruited. Recruitment of fibers follows an orderly pattern. ST fibers are recruited first, and as more force is needed, FT fibers are called into action (Essen, 1978; Gollnick et al., 1973b; Gollnick, Karlsson, Piehl, & Saltin, 1974b; Gollnick, Armstrong, Sembrowich, Shepherd, & Saltin, 1973c). Evidence of recruitment patterns based on glycogen depletion indicates that the pattern of recruitment is first ST fibers, followed by FTa fibers, followed by FTb fibers (Saltin & Gollnick, 1984). Although primarily the ST fibers are involved in low-intensity exercise (Gollnick et al., 1973b; Gollnick et al., 1974b), prolonged submaximal exercise may involve some FT fibers as ST fibers become fatigued. As fatigue increases, more FT fibers continue to be recruited throughout the exercise to exhaustion (Gollnick et al., 1973c). However, in high-intensity exercise requiring forceful contractions, most of the fibers in the muscle may be initially recruited. With little or no reserve of rested fibers to rely on, muscle fatigues rapidly in high-intensity exercise.

Most human skeletal muscles are about 50% ST and 50% FT (Elder, Fense, Sale, & Sutton, 1980; Edgerton, Smith, & Simpson, 1975; Johnson, Polgar, Weightman, & Appleton, 1973; Saltin et al., 1977; Saltin & Gollnick, 1984). One explanation proposed for this mixed fiber composition is that most skeletal muscles are involved in a variety of activities where different characteristics are needed (Saltin et al., 1977). In some muscles, such as the soleus, one fiber type may predominate. The fiber composition of a given muscle varies considerably between individuals and appears to be determined by heredity (Komi et al., 1977). There are apparently no sex differences in muscle fiber composition (Brooke & Engel, 1969; Saltin et al., 1977). There are, however, sex differences in muscle fiber sizes (Brooke & Engel, 1969; Edström & Ekblom, 1972; Edstrom & Nyström, 1969; Saltin et al., 1977.

Men tend to have larger FT and ST fibers than women (Brooke & Engel, 1969). The FT fibers of untrained and trained men are usually larger than their ST fibers (Gollnick, Armstrong, Saubert, Piehl, & Saltin, 1972). In contrast, untrained women have ST fibers that are about the same size or slightly larger than their FT fibers (Brooke & Engel, 1969). The assumed reason for this gender difference is that women are typically less involved in activities requiring forceful contractions and therefore often have poorly developed FT fibers (Saltin et al., 1977). It has been observed that women with handicapped children who must lift extra weight developed FT fibers that were larger than their ST fibers (Brooke & Engel, 1969). Thus, sex differences in fiber size may be due in part to differences in physical activity patterns (Saltin et al., 1977).

Training and Muscle Fiber Composition

Muscle fiber composition may be a factor in successful performance in some activities (Saltin et al., 1977) but apparently is not an important factor in many sports. Successful athletes in most sports have mixed muscle fiber compositions not unlike the average population (Costill et al., 1976a; Costill, Fink, & Pollock, 1976b; Saltin et al., 1977; Saltin & Gollnick, 1984). As previously indicated, this may be explained by the variety of movement requirements for most sports and consequently the need for different fiber types. Nevertheless, there appears to be a relationship between muscle fiber composition and performance in some activities requiring endurance (aerobic power) or power/speed (anaerobic power). Elite athletes in such activities tend to possess a predominance of either ST or FT fibers in the muscles involved in the necessary movements (Saltin et al., 1977; Saltin & Gollnick, 1984). For example, in the vastus lateralis (thigh) muscle, elite endurance runners have a very high percentage of ST fibers, whereas elite sprinters have a very high percentage of FT fibers (Costill et al., 1976b; Saltin et al., 1977; Saltin & Gollnick, 1984). Successful athletes in explosive power events (jumpers, throwers, and weight lifters) do not have an extremely high percentage of FT fibers (Saltin et al., 1977; Saltin & Gollnick, 1984). This may be explained partly by the need for synchronization of muscle fiber contraction in such activities (Saltin et al., 1977). Although women have not been studied as extensively as men, women athletes seem to have muscle fiber compositions (and FT/ST size ratio patterns) similar to men in the same sport (Costill et al., 1976a; Gregor, Edgerton, Perrine, Campion, & Debus, 1979; Nygaard, 1981; Prince, Hikada, & Hagerman, 1977; Saltin et al., 1977).

Based on training studies, muscle fiber composition apparently does not change with strength or endurance training (ST to FT or vice versa) (Gollnick, et al., 1973a; Karlsson, Saltin, Thorstensson, Hulten, & Frith, 1975; Prince, Hikada, & Hagerman, 1976; Saltin et al., 1976; Thorstensson, Sjödin, & Karlsson, 1975; Thorstensson, 1976), although some data suggest an apparent change between FT subgroups (Anderson & Henriksson, 1977;

Henriksson, Jansson, & Schantz, 1980; Jansson & Kaijser, 1977; Jansson, Sjödin, & Tesch, 1978). The evidence of genetic determination of muscle composition along with the studies showing no fiber composition change with training suggest that some elite athletes are born, not made. In some activities, muscle fiber composition could limit elite-level performance. However, muscle fiber composition is obviously not the only factor in successful performance and may, in fact, be relatively unimportant in many sports. Furthermore, possessing a fiber type distribution conducive to distance running, for example, does not, in itself, make the individual a great marathoner. Although he/she may have the potential for success in endurance activities, other factors (training, motivation, cardiovascular fitness, etc.) may be determining factors in success.

Training and Muscle Fiber Size

In contrast to muscle fiber composition, there is considerable evidence that muscle fiber size is affected by physical activity and inactivity (Gollnick et al., 1973a; Saltin et al., 1976). Furthermore, the type of training selectively alters muscle fiber sizes.

Strength training and sprint training can increase the size of both fiber types but may exert a greater effect on FT fibers (Costill et al., 1976a; Saltin et al., 1976; Thorstensson, 1976). For example, male weight lifters have ST and FT muscle fibers that are larger than those of sedentary individuals and endurance athletes (Edström & Ekblom, 1972; Gollnick et al., 1972) and their FT fibers are particularly large. Strength training has been shown to increase the cross-sectional area of FT fibers in several studies (Costill, Coyle, Fink, Lesmes, & Witzman, 1979; Edström & Ekblom, 1972; MacDougall, Ward, Sale, & Sutton, 1977; MacDougall et al., 1979).

Endurance training can produce some hypertrophy in ST fibers with no change in FT fiber size (Gollnick et al., 1973a). Costill, Fink, and Pollock (1976b) found that not only were ST and FT fibers of elite endurance runners significantly larger than those of untrained men, but their ST fibers were 22% larger than their FT fibers. Middle-distance runners and untrained men had equal-sized ST and FT cross-sectional areas. The findings on selective effects of training on muscle fiber types are reasonable, because the fibers activated in training should be the ones to respond to the training stimulus.

Data on fiber sizes of women athletes are much more limited. One reason may be that female athletes have been less trained than male athletes, so effects of strength training on muscle fiber sizes in women have not been well examined. Limited evidence suggests no change in ST or FT fiber sizes of women with 8 weeks of isokinetic training (no changes in fiber sizes were observed in the men either) (Blank & Puhl, 1982). Studies on female athletes indicate that they have smaller muscle fibers than men but larger ST and FT fibers than untrained women (Costill et al., 1976a; Gregor et al., 1979; Nygaard, 1981; Prince et al., 1977). Also, in contrast to sedentary women, who tend to have nearly the same size ST and FT fibers, some female athletes have FT fibers that are larger than their ST fibers (Costill et al., 1976a; Nygaard, 1981), a pattern similar to men. It is reasonable to suggest that the increased physical activity in those female athletes was responsible for increasing the size of both ST and FT fibers. Nevertheless, more information is needed on fiber sizes of female athletes as well as responses of specific fiber types of women to different types of training.

Thus, there is evidence that strength, sprint, and endurance training can selectively alter muscle fiber sizes. The overall effect of training is whole muscle hypertrophy. Although there has been some controversy about the mechanism of muscle hypertrophy (Saltin & Gollnick, 1984) most evidence supports the contention that whole muscle hypertrophy results from an increase in muscle fiber size rather than an increase in fiber number (hyperplasia) (Saltin & Gollnick, 1984). In any case, an increase in muscle size typically results in an increase in muscle strength. Strength is related to the cross-sectional area of the muscle (Ikai & Fukunaga, 1968; Ikai & Fukunaga, 1970) (i.e., the larger the muscle, the greater the force-producing capabilities of that muscle). Although some studies show that training may not alter the relationship between strength and cross-sectional area (Ikai & Fukunaga, 1968; Ikai & Fukunaga, 1970), there is also evidence that strength can increase significantly with very little increase in muscle cross-sectional area (Jansson et al., 1978). Changes in strength with little or no hypertrophy are apparently related to the central nervous system (Saltin & Gollnick, 1984) and the ability to activate all of the motor units. Changes in the ratio of strength to cross-sectional area are most vividly shown by data from strength training studies comparing men and women. For example, Wilmore (1974) found that gains in strength were greater than increases in muscle size in both men and women but that the discrepancy was even greater in women. The gender difference in muscle hypertrophy following weight training programs is presumed to be due to the anabolic (muscle protein deposition) effect of higher endogenous levels of testosterone in men (Wilmore, 1974). The much lower testosterone levels of women may account for the smaller changes in muscle mass in response to weight training as well as their lower percentage of muscle.

It may be assumed from the larger FT fibers of men (both trained and untrained) and the greater increase in FT fiber size with strength training in men that FT fibers are more responsible than ST fibers for total muscle hypertrophy. Possible explanations for sex differences in muscle fiber sizes may be (a) differences in activity patterns between men and women, and (b) the influence of testosterone, particularly on FT fibers.

Muscle Metabolism and Training

ST and FT fibers (Gollnick & Sembrowich, 1977; Gollnick et al., 1973a; Saltin & Gollnick, 1976; Saltin et al., 1977) via increases in substrate storage and/or key enzyme activity (Gollnick & Sembrowich, 1977; Gollnick et al., 1973a;

MacDougall et al., 1977; Saltin et al., 1976; Saltin et al., 1977; Saltin & Gollnick, 1984). With continuous (endurance) training, the increase in SDH activity was greater in ST fibers than in FT fibers (Saltin et al., 1977). With interval training (repeated bouts of high-intensity, short-duration exercise) there was greater SDH activity increase in FT fibers (Saltin et al., 1977), which were presumably used more than in endurance exercise. Thus, the specific fibers activated by the training mode showed increases in potential to use oxygen and produce energy aerobically. Available evidence suggests that endurance training does not significantly alter the glycolytic (anaerobic) potential of muscle fibers (Saltin et al., 1977).

It might be expected that anaerobic training would produce alterations in activity of enzymes involved in anaerobic metabolism resulting in greater potential for anaerobic energy production. Although some small changes have been observed, there is little evidence that strength or sprint training significantly alter anaerobic potential of either fiber type (Costill et al., 1979; Gollnick & Sembrowich, 1977; Gollnick et al., 1972; MacDougall et al., 1979; Saltin et al., 1977).

Muscle Strength/Power/Endurance

Muscle strength, power, and endurance make significant contributions to success in many sports, but their importance depends on the sport. These muscle functions are influenced by muscle fiber composition and the type and amount of training.

Obviously, a larger muscle mass provides an advantage in strength and power activities. Greater strength also contributes to muscle endurance. Women are not as strong as men in most major muscle groups (Fox & Matthews, 1981; Wilmore, 1974) because of their lower muscle mass, which is partly a reflection of training and partly a reflection of biology. There is less sex difference in strength of muscle groups that both men and women use extensively (leg muscles) compared with muscles that women use less than men (upper body) (Brown & Wilmore, 1974; Laubach, 1976; Wilmore, 1974). While differences in absolute strength exist between men and women, these differences diminish when comparisons are made relative to body size (Brown & Wilmore, 1974; Wilmore, 1974).

Men and women respond to strength training similarly (i.e. with the same relative amount and rate of improvement) (Blank & Puhl, 1982; Wilmore, 1974). The result is that men are still stronger than women after strength training. Among athletes in the same sport, men tend to have greater absolute and relative strength than women, but again, the differences diminish when expressed relative to body size (Puhl et al., 1982). In the past, fewer female than male athletes engaged in weight-training programs. Consequently, the gender differences between athletes in the same sport could reflect training differences. Endurance activities do not require a large muscle mass for power. However, muscle strength provides a basis for the necessary muscular endurance. Clearly, weight training is as essential for women as it is for men, particularly for women in sport and competition.

Energy Supply

The human body needs energy for many processes, including muscle contraction. Fuel (energy-carrying molecules of carbohydrate, fat, and protein) is delivered to various cells for either immediate use or stored for later use. These energy-carrying molecules are further broken down within cells to make energy available in a form the cell can use (i.e. a universal energy carrier called ATP—adenosine triphosphate).

Energy Yielding Processes

As the ATP in the cell is used, it can be regenerated in several ways:

1. phosphocreatine (PC) reaction,
2. anaerobic glycolysis, and
3. aerobic metabolism.

PC is a high-energy molecule (like ATP), which acts as an energy reservoir. The reactions using PC to regenerate ATP are anaerobic (no oxygen is needed) as well as alactic (no lactic acid is produced). The amount of ATP that can be provided by this means is limited, enough for a few seconds of contraction. This system is used along with the limited ATP stores when large amounts of energy are used rapidly in activities such as throwing, jumping, kicking, etc. and at the beginning of less intense exercise before the other systems are operating optimally.

Anaerobic glycolysis can use only carbohydrate, does not require oxygen, and results in the end-product lactic acid. Glycolysis is a relatively fast method of producing fairly large amounts of ATP, but it cannot be continued for an extended time. It is used extensively when large amounts of energy are needed in high-intensity exercise that can last from about 30 seconds to 3 min.

Aerobic metabolism can use carbohydrate, fats, and some proteins to regenerate ATP but requires oxygen to do so. This system is far more efficient than anaerobic metabolism in using carbohydrate (glucose). Aerobic metabolism provides most of the energy for exercise covering a wide range of energy requirements—from activities that are easy (rest and light exercise) to those that are moderately strenuous but can be done for a long time (marathon). Activities that can be performed for more than 5 minutes are highly dependent on aerobic metabolism.

All three sources of ATP are used concurrently but in varying proportions depending on the rate of energy required. The rate of energy expenditure depends on exercise intensity and is inversely related to the duration the task can be sustained (i.e., the more intense the task, the higher the rate of energy use, the shorter the duration the task can be sustained, and the more anaerobically dependent it is). Less intense tasks use less energy, can be performed for a longer period, and are more aerobically dependent. Both aerobic and anaerobic metabolism contribute to performance, but their contributions vary depending on the activity. An individual's potential for aerobic and anaerobic energy production sets the limits for performance in various sport activities.

Aerobic Capacity

Because aerobic metabolism uses oxygen, maximal aerobic power (MAP) can be evaluated by measuring the maximal amount of oxygen one can use (maximal oxygen uptake = Max $\dot{V}O_2$). Maximal aerobic power can be limited by respiration (oxygen intake), circulation (oxygen delivery), and/or aerobic metabolism (oxygen utilization for energy production in the muscle). Endurance exercises that last more than 5 min. require a greater ability to use oxygen than activities that last only a couple of minutes. An individual's capacity to use oxygen has limits. Oxygen uptake measured during exercise of progressively increasing intensity will eventually reach the maximum for an individual even though the work and energy requirements continue to increase.

Maximal oxygen uptake is influenced by heredity and training and varies considerably between individuals. In general, larger bodies can use more oxygen. Women have lower absolute maximal oxygen consumption values than men (difference = 56%) (Sparling, 1980), which is in part because of the larger body size of men. However, women also have lower relative MAP values than men (per kg body weight) by about 28% (Sparling, 1980). Because women tend to have smaller hearts and smaller blood volumes per unit of body size as well as lower hemoglobin concentrations than men, their ability to deliver oxygen to working muscles is more limited and may influence their ability to use oxygen. In addition, the higher percentage of body fat of women can account for some of the sex difference in MAP. When values are expressed as $\dot{V}O_2$ per kg fat free weight, the sex difference in MAP diminishes to about 15% (Sparling, 1980). However, these are not practical values, because most physical activities require the athlete to move the entire body weight.

Both male and female endurance trained athletes (i.e., distance runners and cross-country skiiers) have the highest relative MAP values (Bergh, et al., 1978; Drinkwater, 1984; Sharkey, 1984; Wilmore & Brown, 1974). Aerobic training results in similar improvements for men and women (Burke, 1977; Daniels, Kowal, Vogel, & Stauffer, 1979; Eddy, Sparks, & Adelizi, 1977). Training, particularly endurance training, helps reduce the sex difference in relative (per kg body weight) maximal oxygen uptake to about 19% (Drinkwater, 1984). Regardless of the method of expressing MAP, there is considerable overlap between sexes. It is clear that endurance-trained women often have larger relative maximal oxygen uptakes than most men (Bergh et al., 1978; Wilmore & Brown, 1974).

Anaerobic Potential

The more strenuous the exercise, the faster the rate of energy use (ATP/sec) and the more anaerobic metabolism is involved in the energy (ATP) production. Anaerobic metabolism is used extensively, but not exclusively, in high-intensity exercise that can last only a short time (30 sec to 3 min). Thus, one's anaerobic capacity is a limiting factor for high-intensity exercise. Anaerobic metabolism results in the production of lactic acid. Lactic acid measured in the blood after a maximal effort exercise has been used as an indicator of the degree of anaerobiosis that occurred and as an indicator of one's tolerance for anaerobic exercise. Peak blood lactate values for most athletes fall between about 80 and 130 mg% (7 to 12 mM) (unpublished observations). The wide range of values observed is probably due to differences in muscle fiber composition and training. Athletes involved in sports where a high anaerobic capacity is needed (i.e., a half-mile run) usually achieve very high maximal blood lactate values, whereas untrained individuals and athletes in other sports/activities tend to have low or moderate maximal lactate values. Endurance-trained individuals do not necessarily have very high maximal lactic acid values because they do not train as anaerobically as athletes involved in shorter, higher intensity activities. While there is less maximal lactate information available on women than men, generally the information indicates that women, trained or untrained, often have lower maximal lactate values than their male counterparts (Lehman, Keul, Berg, & Stippig, 1981; Puhl, et al. 1982; unpublished observations). These differences could be a reflection of type and/or amount of training.

Anaerobic Threshold

Another measure related to anaerobic capacity is the anaerobic threshold (AT). Lactic acid accumulates at exercise intensities that elicit less than 100% of one's maximal aerobic power. There is an exercise intensity at which the lactic acid level in the blood starts to rise and then increases linearly with increasing exercise intensity (MacDougall, 1979). The point at which blood lactic acid begins to rise is frequently referred to as the AT (Jones & Ehrsam, 1982; Skinner & McLellan, 1980). AT represents the point of transition from primarily aerobic metabolism to a significant amount of anaerobic metabolism. Anaerobic energy production is far less efficient than aerobic, so that beyond this point, performance time is limited. Below AT, lactic acid presumably does not accumulate and the exercise can continue for a long time. Above AT, lactic acid accumulates and performance time becomes limited. High lactic acid levels have been associated with fatigue in nonendurance activities. Therefore, knowledge of the AT may be useful in determining training programs.

One method of identifying AT has been to determine the exercise level at which blood lactate level starts to rise (or goes over 4mM)—the so-called "lactate threshold" (Jones & Ehrsam, 1982), or OBLA (onset of blood lactate accumulation) (Karlsson and Jacobs, 1982). To measure lactic acid during exercise for AT determination requires frequent blood sampling. Consequently, various noninvasive respiratory parameters have been used to try to identify the AT. These respiratory parameters do not always coincide well with the point of blood lactate rise (Skinner & McLellan, 1980; Wasserman, Whipp, Koyal, & Beaver, 1973). Thus, the identification of a breakpoint in certain ventilatory parameters has been called the ventilatory threshold (Jones & Ehrsam, 1982). This value is often adequate to approximate the anaerobic threshold for the purpose of training.

Although terminology is controversial, the so-called anaerobic threshold is important for endurance athletes, because an increase in AT, even when MAP remains constant, can increase the speed (energy output) one can sustain over a long period (Sharkey, 1984). Exercising above AT results in faster glycogen utilization because of the larger amount of anaerobic metabolism, an increased acidity in muscles, and a decrease in the mobilization of lipids (MacDougall, 1979), all of which contribute to a more rapid glycogen depletion. Consequently, pace may decrease earlier in the event and total time may be slower (Sharkey, 1984). In distance runners, performance has been related to the running velocity at AT (Farrell, Wilmore, Coyle, Billing, & Costill, 1979; Sjödin & Jacobs, 1981). AT is not as important for middle distance athletes who compete at intensities above their AT and who need not be concerned about substrate depletion as a limiting factor. For athletes competing in short events, AT is of little consequence. An important factor for the endurance athlete is that AT can be improved by training (Davis & Gass, 1981; Ekblom, Åstrand, Saltin, Stenberg, & Wallstrom, 1968), although it does not always improve (Skinner & McLellan, 1980). Elite endurance athletes have significantly higher ATs than untrained individuals (Hagberg & Coyle, 1983; MacDougall, 1979; Powers, Dodd, Deason, Byrd, & McKnight, 1983). Although Karlsson and Jacobs (1982) have suggested that women may have a lower lactate formation capacity, clearly the observed differences in lactate threshold and peak lactate may be due to differences in levels and/or type of training. Research is very limited and more information is needed.

Some of the observed gender differences in aerobic capacity have a physiological basis that provides an advantage for men. Nevertheless, a portion of the difference may be due to differences in training. Although gender differences in aerobic power may affect performance in middle- and long-distance events, women seem to do well in endurance events. From 1973 to 1983, improvement in the men's marathon record time was 2 min 36 sec vs an improvement for women of 23 min 53 sec (Martin, 1984). In the New York City Marathon, the improvement from 1973 to 1983 was 12 min 55 sec and 30 min 7 sec for men and women, respectively. These differences in improvement reflect women's increased participation in endurance activities and improved training. In short events involving anaerobic metabolism, strength is usually also important for the speed required. It is likely that the strength advantage that men have, rather than a difference in anaerobic metabolism, contributes to gender differences in performance in such events.

Conclusion

There are more physiological similarities than differences between men and women. Biological sex differences may or may not affect performance depending on the sport. Men have several biological advantages that can aid performance in many sports, including endurance activities. Training appears to reduce the gender difference in many physiological characteristics and in performance.

References

Anderson, P., & Henriksson, J. (1977). Training induced changes in the subgroups of human type II skeletal muscle fibers. *Acta Physiologica Scandinavica, 99*, 123-125.

Bergh, U., Thorstensson, A., Sjödin, B., Hulten, B., Piehl, K., & Karlsson, J. (1978). Maximal oxygen uptake and muscle fiber types in trained and untrained humans. *Medicine and Science in Sport and Exercise, 10*, 151-154.

Blank, S., & Puhl, J. (1982). Effect of isokinetic strength training on muscle fiber composition and fiber size in men and women. *Medicine and Science in Sport and Exercise, 14*(2), (Abstract) 112.

Brooke, M., & Engel, W. (1969). The histographic analysis of human muscle biopsies with regard to fiber types. *Neurology* (Minneapolis), **19**, 221-233.

Brown, C.H., & Wilmore, J.H. (1974). The effects of maximal resistance training on the strength and body composition of women athletes. *Medicine and Science in Sport and Exercise, 6*(3), 174-177.

Burke, E.J. (1977). Physiological effects of similar training programs in males and females. *Research Quarterly, 48*, 510-517.

Costill, E.L., Coyle, E.F., Fink, W.F., Lesmes, G.R., & Witzman, F.A. (1979). Adaptations in skeletal muscle following strength training. *Journal of Applied Physiology: Respiratory, Environmental Physiology, 46*, 96-99.

Costill, D.L., Daniels, J., Evans, W., Fink, W., Krahenbuhl, G., & Saltin, B. (1976a). Skeletal muscle enzymes and fiber composition in male and female track athletes, *Journal of Applied Physiology, 40*, 149-154.

Costill, D.L., Fink, W.J., & Pollock, M.L. (1976b). Muscle fiber composition and enzyme activites of elite distance runners. *Medicine and Science in Sport and Exercise, 8*, 96-100.

Daniels, W.L., Kowal, D.M., Vogel, J.A., & Stauffer, R.M. (1979). Physiological effects of military training on male and female cadets. *Aviation Space Environmental Medicine, 50*, 562-566.

Davis, H.A., & Gass, G.C. (1981). The anaerobic threshold as determined before and during lactic acidosis. *European Journal of Applied Physiology, 47*, 141-149.

Drinkwater, B.L. (1984). Women and exercise: physiological aspects. In R.L. Terjung (Ed.), *Exercise and Sport Sciences Reviews*, **12**, 21-51. Lexington, Mass.: The Collomore Press.

Eddy, D.O., Sparks, K.L., & Adelizi, D.A. (1977). The effects of continuous and interval training in women and men. *European Journal of Applied Physiology*, **37**, 83-92.

Edgerton, V.R., Smith, J.L., & Simpson, D.R. (1975). Muscle fiber type populations of human leg muscles. *Histochemistry Journal*, **7**, 259-266.

Edström, L., & Ekblom, B. (1972). Differences in sizes of red and white muscle fibers in vastus lateralis of muscle quadriceps femoris on normal individuals and athletes. *Scandinavian Journal of Clinical Laboratory Investigations*, **30**, 175-181.

Edström, L., & Nyström, B. (1969). Histochemical types and sizes of fibers in normal human muscles. *Acta Neurologica Scandinavica*, **45**, 257-269.

Ekblom, B., Åstrand, P.-O., Saltin, B., Stenberg, J., & Wallström, B. (1968). Effect of training on circulatory response to exercise. *Journal of Applied Physiology*, **24**, 518-525.

Elder, G.C.B., Fense, J., Sale, D., & Sutton, J.R. (1980). Relationship between the fatigue index of the quadriceps and the %FT distribution of the vastus lateralis. *Medicine and Science in Sport and Exercise*, **12**, 143. (Abstract)

Essen, B. (1978). Glycogen depletion of different fiber types in human skeletal muscle during intermittent and continuous exercise. *Acta Physiologica Scandinavica*, **103**, 446-455.

Farrell, P.A., Wilmore, J.H., Coyle, E.P., Billing, J.E., & Costill, D.L. (1979). Plasma lactate accumulation and distance running performance. *Medicine and Science in Sport and Exercise*, **11**, 338-344.

Fleck, S.J. (1983). Body composition of elite American athletes. *American Journal of Sports Medicine*, **11**(6), 398-403.

Fox, E.L., & Matthews, D.K. (1981). *Physiological basis of physical education and athletics*. Philadelphia: W.B. Saunders Co. (pp. 348-394).

Gans, C. (1982). Fiber architecture and muscle function. *Exercise and Sport Science Review*, **10**, 160-207.

Garnett, R.A.F., O'Donovan, M.J., Stephens, J.A., & Taylor, A. (1978). Motor unit organization of human medial gastrocnemius. *Journal of Physiology*, (London), **287**, 33-43.

Gollnick, P.D., Armstrong, R.B., Saltin, B., Saubert IV, C.W., Sembrowich, W.L., & Shepherd, R.E. (1973a). Effect of training on enzyme activity and fiber composition of human skeletal muscle. *Journal of Applied Physiology*, **34**, 107-111.

Gollnick, P.D., Armstrong, R.B., Saubert IV, C.W., Piehl, K., & Saltin, B. (1972). Enzyme activity and fiber composition in skeletal muscle of untrained and trained men. *Journal of Applied Physiology*, **33**, 312-319.

Gollnick, P.D., Armstrong, R.B., Saubert IV, C.W., Sembrowich, W.L., Shepherd, R.E., & Saltin, B. (1973b). Glycogen depletion patterns in human skeletal muscle fibers during prolonged work. *Pflugers Archives*, **344**, 1-12.

Gollnick, P.D., Armstrong, R.B., Sembrowich, W.L., Shepherd, R.E., & Saltin, B. (1973c). Glycogen depletion pattern in human muscle fibers after heavy exercise. *Journal of Applied Physiology*, **34**, 614-618.

Gollnick, P.D., Karlsson, J., Piehl, K., & Saltin, B. (1974a). Selective glycogen depletion in skeletal muscle fibers of man following sustained contractions. *Journal of Physiology*, (London), **241**, 59-67.

Gollnick, P.D., Parsons, D., & Oakley, C.R. Oakley. (1983). Differentiation of fiber types in skeletal muscle from the sequential inactivation of myofibrillar actomyosin ATPase during acid preincubation. *Histochemistry*, **77**, 543-555.

Gollnick, P.D., Piehl, K., & Saltin, B. (1974b). Selective glycogen depletion pattern in human muscle fibers after exercise of varying intensity and at varying pedalling rates. *Journal of Physiology*, (London), **241**, 45-57.

Gollnick, P.D., & Sembrowich, W.L. (1977). Adaptations in Human Skeletal Muscle as a Result of Training. In Amsterdam, E., Wilmore, J.H., & DeMaria, A.N. (Eds.), *Exercise in cardiovascular health and disease*. (pp. 70-94). New York: York Medical Books.

Gregor, R.J., Edgerton, V.R., Perrine, J.J., Campion, D.S., & Debus, C. (1979). Torque-velocity relationships and muscle fiber composition of elite female athletes. *Journal of Applied Physiology: Respiratory Environmental Exercise Physiology*, **47**, 388-392.

Hagberg, J.M., & Coyle, E.F. (1983). Physiological determinants of endurance performance studied in competitive racewalkers. *Medicine and Science in Sport and Exercise*, **15**, 287.

Haymes, E.M., & Dickinson, A.L. (1980). Characteristics of elite male and female ski racers. *Medicine and Science in Sport and Exercise*, **12**(3), 153-158.

Henriksson, J., Jansson, E., & Schantz, P. (1980). Increase in myofibrillar ATPase intermediate skeletal muscle fibers with endurance training of extreme duratin in man. *Muscle Nerve*, **3**, 274. (Abstract)

Ikai, M., & Fukunaga, T. (1968). Calculation of muscle strength per unit cross-sectional area of human muscle by means of ultrasonic measurement. *Int. Z. Angew. Physiol. Einschl. Arbeitphysiol.*, **26**: 26-32.

Ikai, M., & T. Fukunaga. (1970). A study of training effect on strength per unit cross-sectional area of muscle by means of ultrasonic measurement. *Int. Z. Angew. Physiol. Einschl. Arbeitphysiol.*, **28**, 173-180.

Jansson, E., & Kaijser, L. (1977). Muscle adaptation to extreme endurance training in man. *Acta Physiologica Scandinavica*, **100**, 315-324.

Jansson, E., Sjödin, B., & Tesch, P. (1978). Changes in muscle fiber type distribution in man after physical training. *Acta Physiologica Scandinavica,* **104**, 235-237.

Johnson, M.A., Polgar, J., Weightman, D., & Appleton, D. (1973). Data on the distribution of fiber types in thirty-six human muscles. *Journal of Neurological Science,* **18**, 111-129.

Jones, N.L., & Ehrsam, R.E. (1982). The anaerobic threshold. In R.L. Terjung. (Ed.). *Exercise and Sport Sciences Reviews,* **10**, 49-83. Lexington, Mass.: The Collomore Press.

Karlsson, J., & Jacobs, I. (1982). Onset of blood lactate accumulation during muscular exercise as a threshold concept. 1. Theoretical considerations. *International Journal of Sports Medicine,* **3**(4), 190-201.

Karlsson, J.B., Saltin, B., Thorstensson, A., Hulten, B., & Frith, K. (1975). LDH isozymes in skeletal muscles of endurance and strength trained athletes. *Acta Physiologica Scandinavica,* **93**, 150-156.

Komi, P.V., Viitasalo, J.H.T., Havu, M., Thorstensson, A., Sjödin, B., & Karlsson, J. (1977). Skeletal muscle fibers and muscle enzyme activities in monozygous and dizygous twins of both sexes. *Acta Physiologica Scandinavica,* **100**, 385-392.

Laubach, L.L. (1976). Comparative muscular strength of men and women: a review of the literature. *Aviation Space Environmental Medicine,* **47**, 534-542.

Lehman, M., Keul, J., Berg, A., & Stippig, S. (1981). Plasmacatecholamine und metabolische Veraenderungen bei Frauen Waehrend Laufbandergometrie. (Plasma Catecholamine and aerobic-anaerobic capacity in women during graduated treadmill exercise.) *European Journal of Applied Physiology,* **46** (3), 305-315.

MacDougall, J.D. (1979). The anaerobic threshold—its significance to the endurance athlete. *Canadian Journal of Applied Sports Science,* **2**, 13-18.

MacDougall, J.D., Sale, D.G., Moroz, J.R., Elder, G.C.B., Sutton, J.R., & H. Howald. (1979). Mitochondrial volume density in human skeletal muscle following heavy resistance training. *Medicine and Science in Sport and Exercise,* **11**, 164-166.

MacDougall, J.D., Ward, G.R., Sale, D.G., & Sutton, J.R. (1977). Biochemical adaptation of human skeletal muscle to heavy resistance training and immobilization. *Journal of Applied Physiology: Respiratory, Environmental Exercise Physiology,* **43**, 700-703.

Martin, D.E. (1984). Performance of women in endurance sports: interaction of cardiopulmonary with other physiological parameters. *Emory University School of Medicine Gynecology and Obstetrics. Department Bulletin,* **6** (1), 5-20.

Nygaard, E. (1981). Skeletal muscle fiber characteristics in young women. *Acta Physiologica Scandinavica,* **112**, 299-304.

Powers, S.K., Dodd, S., Deason, R., Byrd, R., & McKnight, T. (1983). Ventilatory threshold, running economy, and distance running performance of trained athletes. *Research Quarterly for Exercise and Sport,* **54** (2), 179-182.

Prince, F.P., Hikada, R.S., & Hagerman, F.C. (1976). Human muscle fiber types in power lifters, distance runners and untrained subjects. *Pfleugers Archives,* **363**, 19-26.

Prince, F.P., Hikada, R.S., & Hagerman, F.C. (1977). Muscle fiber types in women athletes and non-athletes. *Pfluegers Archives,* **371**, 161-165.

Puhl, J.L., Case, S., Fleck, S., & Van Handel, P.J. (1982). Physical and physiological characteristics of elite volleyball players. *Research Quarterly for Exercise and Sport,* **53**, 257-262.

Saltin, B., & Gollnick, P.D. (1984). Skeletal muscle adaptability: Significance for metabolism and performance. *Handbook of physiology—skeletal muscle.*

Saltin, B., Henriksson, J., Nygaard, E., Janssen, E., & Anderson, P. (1977). Fiber types and metabolic potentials of skeletal muscles in sedentary man and endurance runners. *Annals of the New York Academy of Science,* **301**, 3-29.

Saltin, B., Nazar, K., Costill, D.L., Stein, E., Jansson, E., Essen, B., & Gollnick, P.D. (1976). The nature of the training response; peripheral and central adaptations to one-legged exercise. *Acta Physiologica Scandinavica,* **96**, 289-305.

Sharkey, B.J. (1984). *Training for cross-country ski racing.* Champaign, IL: Human Kinetics.

Sinning, W.E., Cunningham, L.E., Racaniello, A.P., & Sholes, J.L. (1977). Body composition and somatotype of male and female nordic skiers. *Research Quarterly,* **48** (4), 741-749.

Sjödin, B., & Jacobs, I. (1981) Onset of blood lactic acid and accumulation and marathon running performance. *International Journal of Sports Medicine,* **2**, 26-29.

Skinner, J.S., & McLellan, T.H. (1980). The transition from aerobic to anaerobic metabolism. *Research Quarterly for Exercise and Sport,* **51**, 234-248.

Sparling, P.B. (1980). A meta-analysis of studies comparing maximal oxygen uptake in men and women. *Research Quarterly for Exercise and Sport,* **51**, 542-552.

Thorstensson, A. (1976). Muscle strength, fiber types and enzyme activities in man. *Acta Physiologica Scandinavica,* (Suppl. 443).

Thorstensson, A., Sjödin, B., & Karlsson, J. (1975). Enzyme activities and muscle strength after ''sprint training'' in man. *Acta Physiologica Scandinavica,* **94**, 313-318.

Wasserman, K., Whipp, B.J., Koyal, S.N., & Beaver, W.L. (1973). Anaerobic threshold and respiratory gas exchange during exercise. *Journal of Applied Physiology, 35,* 236-243.

Wilmore, J.H. (1974). Alterations in strength, body composition and anthropometric measurements consequent to a 10-week weight training program. *Medicine and Science in Sports,* **6** (2), 133-138.

Wilmore, J.H. (1976). *Athletic training and physical fitness.* Boston: Allyn and Bacon.

Wilmore, J.H. (1979). The application of science to sport: Physiological profiles of male and female athletes. *Canadian Journal of Applied Sport Science,* **4,** 103-115.

Wilmore, J.H., & Brown, C.H. (1974). Physiological profiles of women distance runners. *Medicine and Science in Sports,* **6,** 178-181.

3 The Psychology of the Female Runner

Dorothy V. Harris

Penn State University

No physical activity to date has ever generated more enthusiasm and interest than running. It is difficult to determine the exact number of runners in the world; however, in the United States estimates between 20 to 30 million have been made. Of these, approximately 20% are female. During the surge in participation, considerable attention has been directed to the physiological and medical aspects of jogging and running. There is generally a relative lack of data and information about the mental and emotional aspects of running.

Interest in the mental well-being associated with vigorous exercise is not new. The Greek ideal of sound body, sound mind is well known. Only recently have efforts been made to systematically address the relationship of exercise and well-being. The universal testimony of regular exercisers is that they "feel better." Regular runners report that running makes them feel better (Callen, 1983; Carmack & Martens, 1979; Jorgenson & Jorgenson, 1979; Nowlis & Greenberg, 1979). Several investigators have found that marathon runners (Gondola & Tuckman, 1982; Morgan & Pollock, 1977; Wilson, Morley, & Bird, 1980), racers (Joesting, 1982), and joggers (Wilson et al., 1980) tend to report more positive moods on the Profile of Mood State (POMS) in depression fatigue, confusion, tension, and anger, and higher scores on vigor than nonexercising controls. Carmack and Martens (1979) reported that runners who missed their regular exercise experienced more bad moods, guilt, irritability, depression, and sluggishness.

A well-known female runner sums up the runners' self-reports and observations in this manner, "I'm always amused when nonrunners express amazement at my daily running and admire my supposedly tremendous willpower, which enables me to drive myself so hard. Actually, I have very little willpower and am basically a hedonist. I wouldn't run if I didn't like it. In fact, if I take more than a few days off now, I have physical withdrawal symptoms like any addict . . . headache, nervousness ('bitchiness,' my husband elaborates helpfully), insomnia, and constipation. I plunge back into running with tremendous relief and an exhilarating 'high.' This is a common phenomenon among long-distance runners," (Callen, 1983; 133-134.).

Frequent references are made throughout the literature to "runner's high," "second wind," "altered state," and "feel better" experience as a phenomenon associated with long-distance running. Despite the wealth of anecdotal evidence to support the idea that endurance running produces unusual and interesting mental phenomena, to date no psychometric correlates have been discovered for this experience. However, the research and literature available would seem to support the idea that exercise has a somatopsychic effect (Harris, 1973).

Personality and Self-Perceptions

One of the first studies examining behavioral traits of marathoners was completed by Morgan and Costill (1972), who reported that these runners represent a "special breed." Male marathoners scored much lower than the normative group on anxiety and extroversion variables. Mikel (1983) gave the Eysenck Personality Inventory (EPI) to 310 adult runners (94 female) and observed that female runners were significantly more extroverted than males. Generally females tend to score lower on extroversion than males. Mikel suggested that her findings may indicate that the more introverted female shuns the activity of running because the visibility is so high. More recently Ismail (1984) demonstrated that adult males became more extroverted and less neurotic as their physical fitness improved with regular exercise. According to Morgan (1978), elite runners are quite extroverted.

Other studies focusing on the psychological variables of long-distance runners indicate that runners are more intelligent (Burdick & Zloty, 1973; Valliant, Bennie & Valliant, 1981) and imaginative (Farge & Hartung, 1978). Valliant et al (1981) found that runners were more self-sufficient and tender-minded and Farge and Hartung (1978) reported that both joggers and distance runners were more outgoing, intelligent, enthusiastic, venturesome, imaginative, astute, and self-sufficient than the general population. Jerome and Valliant (1983) compared cross-country skiers and marathon runners on Cattell's 16 Personality Factor Inventory and reported many similarities. The runners appeared more intelligent and tough-minded, however, they were significantly older. Jerome and Valliant (1983) suggested that it is possible that prolonged exposure to endurance activities maximizes one's predisposition to a specific behavioral trait or that as one matures, personality traits become more pronounced.

In a psychological study of 50 sub-3-hour marathoners, Gontang, Clitsome and Kostrubala (1977), using the Myers-Briggs Type Indicator (MBTI), reported that there were twice as many introverts as extroverts among their population. Further, 96% of the marathoners had college-level education or better (which would explain the greater intelligence found among marathoners by other investigators).

In one of the first studies completed on female marathoners, Harris and Jennings (1977) examined the personal attributes of scholastic and club runners. The ages of the scholastic group ranged from 14 to 23, while the club group's ages ranged from 26 to 59. Using the Personal Attributes Questionnaire (PAQ), the runners were classified according to their behavioral frame of reference: androgynous, masculine, feminine, or undifferentiated.

When the relationship of the PAQ classification and self-esteem was examined, those runners who were classified as androgynous or masculine displayed significantly higher self-esteem. Traditionally it has been assumed that females who perceive themselves as being more closely aligned with typical masculine behavior would display dissonance and lower self-esteem. One can conclude that either marathon running improves self-esteem or that females who have higher self-esteem are more likely to engage in marathon running.

Table 1 PAQ Classification of Runners*

Sample	Femininity		Masculinity	
	n	% [a]	n	% [a]
	Undifferentiated		*Masculine*	
Below Median				
Total Sample	14	20.6	19	27.9
Club	7	20.6	12	35.3
Scholastic	7	20.6	7	20.6
	Feminine		*Androgynous*	
Above Median				
Total Sample	12	17.6	23	33.8
Club	5	14.7	10	29.4
Scholastic	7	20.6	13	38.2

* Club total n = 34: Scholastic total n = 34.
[a] Percentages are adjusted frequencies.

Motivation, Commitment and Addiction

Ten long-distance female runners, aged 25 to 51 were interviewed by Hendry (1978). Health, pleasure, self-expression, and appearance were the major motives for running. Carmack and Martens (1979), in the process of developing a Commitment to Running Scale (CR) tested 75 female and 250 male runners. A significantly greater proportion of females reported that they experienced discomfort when they missed a run despite the fact that their perceived "addiction" score was not significantly different from the males' score. This was an unexpected finding, because the males had a higher score on the commitment to running. It was assumed that the greater the commitment to running, the greater the discomfort when a run was missed.

A survey (Harris, 1981a) of 409 runners' (132 female) perceptions of the benefits of running revealed that the major reasons given for running were feeling better physically and psychologically. Females reported more frequently than males that they started and continued to run to become more fit, to lose or control weight, to look better, or because they had friends and relatives who were running. Females were also more likely to report they felt guilty when they missed their regular run.

In a later study Harris (1981b) surveyed 156 women runners to discover why they were participating in what was once a stereotyped masculine activity and what they perceived the psychological and behavioral effects of running to be. These women runners generally displayed positive views of running and indicated that they received support for running from others and would encourage other women to run. They indicated that running made them feel significantly stronger, happier, more relaxed, better about themselves, and more attractive, energetic, and feminine. They also reported that they felt guilty, fatter, depressed, tense, and less energetic when they did not run. Harris (1981b) concluded that it appears that women runners view running as a positive experience that enhances their femininity rather than increases their masculinity.

The mental and emotional aspects of long-distance running were surveyed among 424 runners (121 female) by Callen (1983). Many of those surveyed started running to improve their health; however, almost all noted psychological benefits such as relief of tension, improved self-image, and better moods. Two thirds of them indicated they had experienced a "runner's high" and about one half of them had experienced trance-like states, enhanced visual imagery, and creative episodes during some of the runs. More women than men claimed that running relieved depression and produced better moods.

The positive psychological benefits of long-distance running have been documented to the extent that Glasser (1976) has described the experience as a "positive addiction." Further, most runners indicate that they feel less well without their regular run. This response, along with the persistence of the running habit despite illness, stress fractures, inclement weather, etc., has led to viewing the running habit among many as "negative addiction" (Morgan, 1979). Morgan says one is addicted when he or she requires daily exercise to cope and believes he or she cannot live without daily exercise. A second characteristic of the addicted runner is, if deprived of exercise, various withdrawal symptoms are manifested. Exercise addicts who are forced by injury or some other reason to stop running often become depressed, anxious, and extremely irritable. These symptoms are accompanied by a host of other somatic manifestations such as restlessness, insomnia, fatigue, muscle tension, constipation, etc. Exercise addicts continue to run when injured and give their daily run higher priority than job, family, or friends. They often run to the point where overuse injuries produce near-crippling effects. When the pain becomes intolerable, they search for the perfect shoe, sports medicine doctor, drug, pain killer, or psychological strategy that will enable them to continue to run. The number of runners that would actually be categorized as "negatively addicted" is not known; however, sufficient evidence is being generated to suggest that negative addiction in runners is becoming a problem.

The solution to this problem appears simple: Runners must keep their exercise programs in perspective, controlling the running experience rather than letting running control them. Goal setting, learning how to read personal body signals to develop greater self-awareness, developing greater self-awareness, and developing interests beyond exercise help to keep the responses to regular exercise in the positive column. Keep in mind that running is a means to an end—enhanced health and well being.

The Effects of Exercise on Depression

Using an experimental design to study the effects of exercise on depression Greist, Klein, Eischens, and Faris (1978) randomly assigned 28 subjects to one of three treatment groups: (1) ten sessions of time-limited psychotherapy; (2) time-unlimited psychotherapy; or (3) running with a group leader for 30 to 65 minutes three times per week. All treatments were conducted over a 10-week period. The subjects were 13 men and 15 women who scored above the 50th percentile on the SCL-90 depression scale. The eight subjects assigned to the running treatment had at least as much improvement in their levels of depression as those under the two psychotherapy treatments.

Rueter, Harris, and Mutrie (1984) conducted a study similar to that of Greist et al. (1978). Eighteen subjects who had sought help for depression at a mental health clinic of a large university were randomly assigned to either a counseling therapy group or a group combining psychotherapy with running three times per week. The group that combined running with psychotherapy improved significantly more than the counseling-only group over a 10-week period.

This approach was expanded by Fremont (1983), who randomly assigned 49 depressed volunteers to three groups: (1) cognitive therapy 1 hr per week; (2) running with a group leader for 20 min three times per week; or (3) counseling 1 hr per week combined with running 20 min three times per week. At the end of ten weeks of treatment Fremont (1983) found that all three treatments produced equal and significant improvements in depression.

Depression levels of marathoners who ran between 6 and 20 miles six to seven days a week were compared with those of joggers who averaged 1

Table 2 Pre- and Post-Scores on the Beck Depression Inventory (BDI)

Subjects	Totals	Means	SD
Running Group (n = 9)			
Pre-BDI	207	23.00	7.58
Post-BDI	46	5.10	4.75
Non-Running Group (n = 9)			
Pre-BDI	208	23.10	11.02
Post-BDI	167	18.56	7.70

Note. From "Running as an adjunct to counseling therapy in the treatment of depression," by M.A. Rueter, D.V. Harris, and N. Mutrie, 1984, unpublished manuscript.

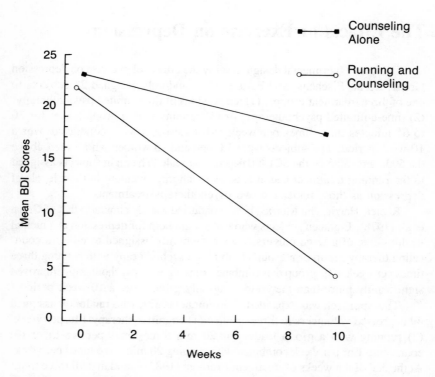

Figure 1. Running and counseling therapy versus counseling alone

Note. From "Running as an adjunct to counseling therapy in the treatment of depression," by M.A. Rueter, D.V. Harris, and N. Mutrie, 1984, Unpublished manuscript.

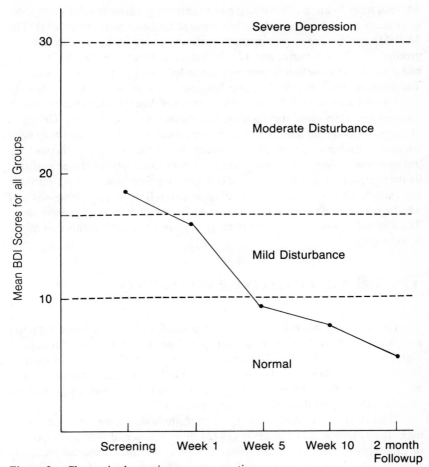

Figure 2.   Change in depression scores over time

Note.   From ''The separate and combined effects of cognitively based counseling and aerobic exercise for the treatment of mild and moderate depression,'' by J. Fremont, 1983, Unpublished doctoral dissertation, the Pennsylvania State University.

to 2 miles three to five days a week and with nonexercisers who had not participated in any physical activity during the last year. Wilson, Morley and Bird (1980) found that marathoners and joggers were significantly less depressed than nonexercisers as measured by the POMS.

Slow long-distance running appears to work equally well for children. Shipman (1984) studied 56 children, 34 of whom were on some type of psychotropic medication for treatment of aggressiveness, impulsiveness, and hyperkinesis. After 18 weeks (six weeks of training followed by 12 weeks of running a maximum of 45 min four times per week) the major finding was that psychotropic medication can be reduced in emotionally disordered children who run long distances. Disturbing and sometimes permanent side effects from these medications have stimulated the desire to find alternative treatments. The 34 children who were on psychotropic medication were further divided into two groups, 17 who ran more, and 17 who ran less. Ten of the 12 children who had a significant reduction in their medication fell into the "ran more" category. The more a child ran, the less psychotropic medication was prescribed.

Overall the design and nature of the studies of depression among exercisers and nonexercisers make it difficult to determine the causal factors. The types of people who are attracted to exercise, the expectancies individuals may have when they embark on a running program, or a host of other variables may influence the findings. However, the research and anecdotal evidence available to date suggest that runners are less depressed than nonrunners. Further, individuals who are diagnosed as being moderately or mildly depressed and who begin a running program display a significant reduction in their depression. The available evidence does not identify any specific mechanisms that might be operating.

The Effects of Exercise on Anxiety

Exercise may be truly nature's best tranquilizer; the literature supports a reduction in both state and trait anxiety and decreased tension with regular vigorous exercise. In one of the first studies reporting behavioral responses to exercise Baekeland (1970) observed that habitual runners who were asked not to exercise for a month had increased sexual tension, anxiety, a need to be with others, and disturbed sleeping patterns.

The effects of 10 weeks of jogging were studied, among other variables, by Folkins, Lynch, and Gardener (1972). Both males and females improved in fitness; however, only the women demonstrated psychological changes; namely, decreased depression and anxiety and increased self-confidence.

Tooman, Harris, and Mutrie (1984) examined the effect of running and its deprivation on anxiety and mood. The beneficial effects of running were supported indirectly when two groups of runners, competitive (n = 20) and recreational (n = 20) with similar running histories and capabilities, were asked not to run for two days while anxiety and moods were monitored. The testing covered a four-day period with the runners reporting for the testing before a regular run. Measures on the POMS and the State-Trait Anxiety Inventory (STAI) were taken before and after the run and the subsequent two days without running. On Day 4 the subjects were asked to resume their regular running pattern and report for testing after the run.

The POMS and STAI scores were subjected to a 2 (competitive vs recreational runners) × 5 (testing sessions) analysis of variance with repeated measures. There was a significant main effect for type of runner on state anxiety $F (1,38) = 6.102$, $p < .05$, with the competitive runners being significantly lower. A significant main effect on the anger subscale of the POMS was also observed with the competitive runners being significantly less angry F $(1,38) = 5.273, p < .05$. By comparing the means on the dependent measures from the prerun and postrun on Day 1, an acute response was observed. One running session significantly reduced feelings of anxiety, tension, depression, anger, and confusion for all runners.

The results of this study also demonstrated that depriving regular runners of two days of running increased state anxiety levels, tension, and confusion. Further, the results suggest that the positive effects of a single running session lasts for at least one day without exercise. Berger (1984) has also reported the acute and chronic effects of swimming by demonstrating reduced state and trait anxiety levels.

Table 3   Pre- and Post-Run Mood Scores (POMS) For Runner ($n = 40$)

Mood	Pre-Run	Post-Run
Anger	4.73	1.95*
Confusion	5.80	4.10*
Depression	6.18	3.70*
Fatigue	6.43	5.33
Tension	7.45	3.25*
Vigor	17.33	18.48
State Anxiety (STAI)	34.70	30.52*

*$p < .01$
Note. "The effect of running and its deprivation on muscle tension, mood, and anxiety," by M.E. Tooman, D.V. Harris, and N. Mutrie, 1982, unpublished manuscript.

Mood Changes with Exercise

Using the POMS to assess changes in moods in both acute and chronic exercisers, a series of studies have produced similar findings. Several investigators have found that marathon runners (Gondola & Tuckman, 1982; Morgan & Pollock, 1977; Wilson, Morley & Bird, 1979), racers (Joesting, 1981) and joggers (Wilson et al., 1979) tend to report lower scores on the POMS than nonexercising controls. Runners display significantly less depression, fatigue, confusion, tension, and anger and more vigor.

When competitive runners were compared to recreational runners, Tooman, Harris and Mutrie (1984) found that competitive runners had more positive moods than recreational runners on all six POMS subscales; anger was the only mood state to show a statistically significant difference, with the recreational runners displaying more anger. In this study the runners were tested five times over four days: before and after a regular run on Day 1, without running on Days 2 and 3 and after a run on Day 4. The more positive mood profile that described the runners after their initial run on Day 1 was maintained into the second day without another run. However, by the second day with no running most of the mood indicators had returned to the prerun mood profile of Day 1. These changes were all significantly different from the postrun profile of Day 1. The single exception to this pattern was that vigor was significantly lower than at the prerun stage on Day 1.

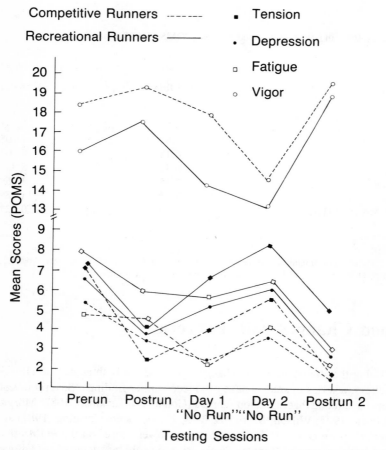

Figure 3.   Patterns of tension, depression, vigor and fatigue for competitive and recreational runners.

Note. From ''The effect of running and its deprivation on muscle tension, mood, and anxiety,'' by M.E. Tooman, D.V. Harris, and N. Mutrie, 1982, Unpublished manuscript.

On Day 4 the subjects resumed their regular exercise pattern. All mood variables showed a significant change in a positive direction, with fatigue significantly lower than at the postrun stage of Day 1.

Mood changes over 10 weeks were also monitored by Fremont (1983), who used the POMS. He reported that depression, tension, anger, confusion, and frustration dropped significantly over the 10 weeks of using jogging, psychotherapy, and a combination of the two. Vigor increased significantly across all groups as well.

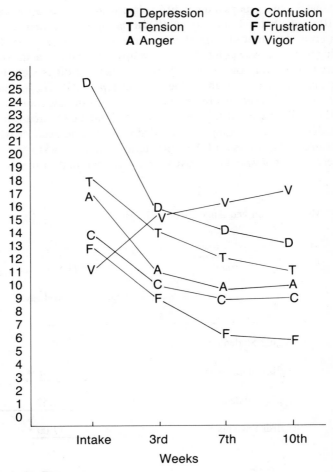

Figure 4. Summary of POMS

Note. From "The separate and combined effects of cognitively based counseling and aerobic exercise for the treatment of mild and moderate depression," by J. Fremont, 1983, Unpublished doctoral dissertation, The Pennsylvania State University.

The effect of regular exercise (jogging 10 weeks, three times per week) on mood (POMS) was compared to an English class who served as controls (Mutrie & Harris, 1984). The experimental group was enrolled in a jogging class; the control group was not involved in any exercise program. Both groups were tested on the POMS at the beginning, midway through, and at the end of the 10 weeks.

A MANOVA showed a significant group (jogging, English) X time (beginning, midway, end) interaction, $F(2,25) = 4.01$, $p < .03$. The subsequent univariate ANOVA's showed two of the variables to have significant interaction effects, anger, $F(2,47) = 3.48$, $p < .04$ and tension, $F(2,51)$ 3.63, $p < .04$. Follow-up tests on the simple effects of the group X time interactions showed that the two groups did not differ significantly at the beginning or end of the 10 weeks but did differ ($p < .05$) at the midway testing period. The English class also showed a significant increase in anger ($p < .05$) from the beginning to the midway point. The two groups did not differ at the beginning of the term on the tension variable; however, they did differ significantly at both the midpoint and at the end of the ten weeks ($p < .05$). The jogging group showed a significant decrease in tension from beginning to end ($p < .05$), while the English group showed a significant increase in tension at the midpoint. These findings suggest that students who exercise while they are adjusting to the stresses of their first term of university study cope more effectively than those who do not have exercise as a part of their regular routine.

Table 4   Mean Tension and Anger Scores (POMS)

Mood	Group	Time of Term		
		Begin	Midway	End
Anger	Jogging Students ($n = 14$)	9.21	6.57	6.86
	English Students ($n = 14$)	7.36	13.36[a]*	8.98
Tension	Jogging Students	10.50	7.57	6.79[a]
	English Students	12.36	17.00[a]*	13.14*

* p .04
[a] p .04

Note. From "Comparison of mood changes in jogging and English students," by N. Mutrie and D.V. Harris, 1984, unpublished manuscript.

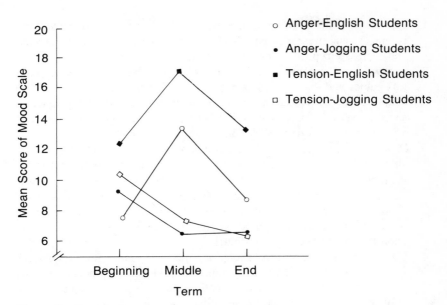

Figure 5.   Pattern of anger and tension scores (POMS)

Note. From "Comparison of mood changes in jogging and English students," by N. Mutrie and D.V. Harris, 1984, Unpublished manuscript.

In summarizing the research and the anecdotal evidence it appears that long-distance running serves as an effective treatment to moderate and mild depression. Anxiety levels decrease with regular endurance exercise and positive moods are enhanced and accompanied by a perception of more vigor. Further, insomnia tends to be reduced with regular endurance exercise. Females appear to have more to gain by becoming involved in regular endurance exercise because they appear to have more problems with depression, anxiety, and insomnia than do males. In short, females have everything to gain (except weight) and nothing to lose (except weight) when they incorporate endurance activities into their life-styles.

Theoretical Hypotheses That May Add Insight and Understanding

At this point in the knowledge and understanding of the effects of endurance exercise on psychological factors only the association of exercise with decreases in depression and anxiety and increased positive moods can be made. The causal mechanisms are not known. However, there are several hypotheses that have been proposed by Morgan (1984) and others.

1 *Distraction.* This hypothesis proposes that distraction or time out from stimuli causing stress is responsible for the reduction in anxiety, depression, and increase in positive moods rather than the exercise.

2 *Rhythmicity.* For centuries it has been observed that rocking quiets restless babies and that music has a quieting effect. It is hypothesized here that the rhythm produced by such activities as running, swimming, cycling, aerobic exercise, etc., may "quiet" the central nervous system in such a manner that positive psychological effects occur.

3 *Dependence or Addiction.* The observation that some individuals are more susceptible to becoming addicted to substances than others has generated the hypothesis that some individuals may become addicted to exercise more easily than others. Most runners who exercise on a regular basis would probably prefer to be considered exercise *dependent* rather than exercise *addicted.* This dependency or addiction may be a psychobiological phenomenon that has yet to be identified.

4 *Elevated Body Temperature.* Increasing the body temperature to produce a variety of effects viewed as therapeutic has been the practice of many who use heat, steam rooms, sauna baths, and the like. Elevating the body temperature to the point of sweating may be necessary to produce therapeutic effects.

5 *Endorphin Secretion.* One of the more popular hypotheses posed in the last few years has suggested that exercise-induced euphoria is a result of increased plasma beta-endorphin levels. There is evidence to suggest that endorphin levels do increase in response to physical stress such as endurance exercise. This hypothesis may be related to the increase in monoamines such as norepinephrine and serotonin, which in turn trigger additional neurotransmitters secreted in the brain such as the beta-endorphins.

Summary

Both acute and chronic physical exercise of a vigorous and endurance nature have improved psychological well-being. However, at this point it is not clear why this type of exercise is associated with improved affective states. Further research is needed to identify the mechanisms that produce these changes. In the meantime, thousands of runners have discovered that they feel better with regular vigorous exercise and will continue to follow that routine without waiting for all the evidence to be reported.

References

Baekeland, F. Exercise deprivation. (1970). *Archives of General Psychiatry,* **22**, 365-369.

Berger, B. (1984, April). *Swimmers report less stress.* Paper presented at the NIMH Workshop on Coping with mental stress: The potential and limits of exercise intervention. Bethesda, MD.

Burdick, J.A. & Zloty, R.B. (1973). Wakeful heart rate, personality and performance, a study of distance runners. *Journal of Sports Medicine and Physical Fitness, 13,* 17-25.

Callen, K. (1983). Mental and emotional aspects of long-distance running. *Psychosomatics, 24,* 133-151.

Carmack, M.A., & Martens, R. (1979). Measuring commitment to running: A survey of runners' attitudes and mental states. *Journal of Sports Psychology, 1,* 25-43.

Farge, E.J. & Hartung, G.H. (1978). Personality and physiological traits in middle-age runners and joggers. *Journal of Gerontology, 32,* 541-548.

Folkins, C.H., Lynch, S., & Gardener, M.M. (1972). Psychological fitness as a function of physical fitness. *Archives of Physical Medicine and Rehabilitation, 53,* 503-508.

Fremont, J. (1983). *The separate and combined effects of cognitively based counseling and aerobic exercise for the treatment of mild and moderate depression.* Unpublished doctoral dissertation, The Pennsylvania State University.

Glasser, W. (1976). *Positive addiction.* New York: Harper Row.

Gondola, J.C., & Tuckman, B.W. (1982). Psychological mood state in "average" marathon runners. *Perceptual and Motor Skills, 55,* 1295-1300.

Gontag, A., Clitsome, T., & Kostrubala, T. (1977). A psychological study of 50 sub-3-hour marathoners. *Annals of the New York Academy of Sciences, 301,* 1020-1028.

Greist, J.H., Klein, M.H., Eischens, R.R., & Faris, J.T. (1978). Running out of depression. *The Physician and Sports Medicine, 6,* (12), 49-50.

Harris, D.V. (1973). *Involvement in sport: A somatopsychic rationale for physical activity.* Philadelphia: Lea Febiger.

Harris, D.V. & Jennings, S.E. (1977). Self-perceptions of female distance runners. *Annals of the New York Academy of Sciences, 301,* 808-815.

Harris, M.B. (1981a). Runner's perceptions of the benefits of running. *Perceptual and Motor Skills, 52,* 153-154.

Harris, M.B. (1981b). Women runners' views of running. *Perceptual and Motor Skills, 53,* 395-402.

Hendry, C.H. (1978, Summer). Motivation and female distance runners. *Running, 3,* 16-17.

Ismail, A.H. (1984, April). Psychological effects of exercise in the middle years. Paper presented at NIMH Workshop on Coping with mental stress: The potential and limits of exercise intervention. Bethesda, MD.

Jerome, W.C. & Valliant, P.M. (1983). Comparison of personalities between marathon runners and cross-country skiers. *Perceptual and Motor Skills, 56,* 35-38.

Joesting, J. (1981). Running and depression. *Perceptual and Motor Skills, 52,* 442.

Jorgenson, C.B., & Jorgenson, D.E. (1979). Effect of running on perception of self and others. *Perceptual and Motor Skills, 48*, 242.

Mikel, K.V. (1983). Extraversion in adult runners. *Perceptual and Motor Skills, 57*, 143-146.

Morgan, W.P. (1978). The mind of the marathoner. *Psychology Today, 11*, 38-49.

Morgan, W.P. (1979). Negative addiction in runners. *Physician and Sportsmedicine, 7*, 57-70.

Morgan, W.P. (1984, April). *Affective beneficience of vigorous physical activity.* Paper presented at the NIMH Workshop on Coping with Mental Stress: The potential and limits of exercise intervention. Bethesda, MD.

Morgan, W.P., & Costill, D.L. (1972). Psychological characteristics of the marathon runner. *Journal of Sports Medicine and Physical Fitness, 12*, 42-46.

Morgan, W.P., & Pollock, M.L. (1977). Psychologic characterization of the elite distance runner. *Annals of the New York Academy of Sciences, 301*, 382-403.

Mutrie, N., & Harris, D.V. (1984). *Comparison of mood changes in jogging and English students.* Unpublished manuscript, The Pennsylvania State University, University Park, PA.

Nowlis, D.P., & Greenberg, N. (1979). Empirical description of effects of exercise on mood. *Perceptual Motor Skills, 49*, 1001-1002.

Rueter, M.A., Harris, D.V., & Mutrie, N. (1984). *Running as an adjunct to counseling therapy in the treatment of depression.* Unpublished manuscript, The Pennsylvania State University, University Park, PA.

Shipman, W.M. (1984). Emotional and behavioral effects of long-distance running on children. In Sachs, M.L., & Buffone, G.W. (Eds.) *Running as therapy* (pp. 125-137). Lincoln: University of Nebraska Press.

Tooman, M.E., Harris, D.V., & Mutrie, N. (1982). *The effect of running and its deprivation on muscle tension, mood and anxiety.* Unpublished manuscript, The Pennsylvania State University, University Park, PA.

Valliant, P.M., Bennie, F.A.B., & Valliant, J.J. (1981). Do marathoners differ from joggers in personality profile: Sports psychology approach. *Journal of Sport Medicine and Physical Fitness, 21*, 62-67.

Wilson, V.E., Morley, N.C., & Bird, E.I. (1980). Mood profiles of marathon runners, joggers, and nonexercisers. *Perceptual and Motor Skills, 5*, 117-118.

4 Biomechanics of Distance Running: A Focus on Women

Anne E. Atwater

University of Arizona

In the 1977 proceedings of a New York Academy of Sciences conference on "The Marathon," Nelson, Brooks, and Pike (1977) stated that little information was available on the biomechanics of female distance runners. Even though participation in distance running by girls and women has increased dramatically since 1977, there is still a paucity of scientific data describing the biomechanical factors associated with skilled performance in this group of athletes. This paper reviews selected biomechanical literature on running speed, stride length, stride rate, and angular position-time profiles of arm motion, with special reference to the performance of female distance runners.

Running Speed, Stride Length, and Stride Rate

To place the accomplishments of women marathon runners in perspective, improvements in world record times for men and women can be compared over the past 20 years. The men's record in 1964 was 2:12:11, only 3 min 51 sec slower than Alberto Salazar's current world record time of 2:08:13 set in 1981. In 1964 the competitive marathon was still relatively new to women, and their world record time was 3:19:33. The 1983 current world record of 2:22:43 by Joan Benoit represents an improvement of almost 1 hr over the 1964 record. In fact, 267 women qualified for the first Women's Olympic Marathon Trials by achieving a 1983 marathon time under 2:51.16.

Most experienced marathon runners have developed a good sense of pace and try to maintain a relatively even speed throughout a race. If it were assumed that a runner could maintain a constant pace for 26.22 miles, the running speeds listed in Table 1 (expressed in min/mile and in m/s) would be required to produce the marathon times listed in the left-hand column.

Table 1 Selected Marathon Times and Associated Steady-State Running Speeds

Marathon Time (hr, min, sec)	Min/Mile	m/s
2:20:45	5.37	5.00
2:22:43*	5.45	4.93
2:37:18	6.00	4.47
2:50:25	6.50	4.13
3:03:31	7.00	3.83
3:20:59	7.67	3.50
3:54:28	8.94	3.00

*Women's World Record, Joan Benoit, 4-18-83.

Running speed is determined by the product of two variables, stride length and stride rate. However, the relationship between each of these variables and running speed has been shown by several investigators to be a nonlinear relationship (Dillman, 1975; Luhtanen & Komi, 1978; Saito, Kobayashi, Miyashita, & Hoshikawa, 1974). As running speed increases at lower velocities (3.0 to 6.5 m/s), larger increments are made in stride length than in stride rate. At higher running speeds (6.5 to 10+ m/s), proportionately greater increases are made in stride rate, whereas stride length changes relatively little and may even decrease slightly at maximal speeds. For skilled male runners, the critical speed after which changes in stride rate are generally greater than changes in stride length appears to be approximately 6.5 m/s (Dillman, 1975). It is possible that this critical speed may be somewhat lower than 6.5 m/s for female runners.

Biomechanical comparisons were made by Nelson et al. (1977) between a group of 21 elite American female distance runners and a group of 10 university male distance runners. Both groups of subjects were filmed while running overground at seven equally spaced velocities ranging from 4.83 m/s to 6.74 m/s. At all seven velocities the female runners had significantly shorter strides and higher stride rates than did the men. The women as a group were significantly shorter than the men, which explains their need to take shorter but more frequent steps to maintain the same absolute velocity as the male runners. When stride length was expressed as a percent of each subject's height, the female runners had significantly longer relative stride lengths (108%) than the male runners (104%) across all running speeds. On the basis of these measurements, Nelson et al. concluded that the females appeared to be overstriding when compared with the male model.

To compensate for individual differences in maximum running speed, Nelson et al. conducted a second analysis in which relative velocities of 60%, 70%, 80%, and 90% of each runner's maximum velocity were used. This approach reduced, but did not eliminate, the differences between male and female distance runners on the variables of stride length (absolute and relative), stride rate, and the temporal components of stride time.

The possibility that some female runners may overstride when running alone or with a taller companion has a potential link to running injuries. Specifically, stress fractures of the inferior pubic ramus and/or periosteal reaction in the area of adductor muscle insertion on the femur were diagnosed in 67 females (average height 63.7 in.) and three males (average height 65 in.) in their first 12 weeks of military training (Ozburn & Nichols, 1981). All patients related their symptoms to marching, and most described "taking giant steps all day" to keep up with their platoon.

Stress fractures of the inferior pubic ramus in competitive and recreational runners are less common than stress fractures of the tibia, fibula, and metatarsals (Prescott, 1983; Tehranzadeh, Kurth, Elyaderani, & Bowers, 1982). However, pelvic stress fractures have been reported to occur with greater frequency in female runners than in male runners (Latshaw, Kantner, Kalenak, Baum, & Corcoran, 1981; Pavlov, Nelson, Warren, Torg, & Burstein, 1982; Prescott, 1983). Although the relationships of stride length, other aspects of running technique, and even female pelvic anatomy are indeterminate to the incidence of pelvic stress fractures, this topic deserves further investigation.

Angular Position-Time Profiles of Arm Motion

Despite the fact that running has been the focus of numerous biomechanical studies, the motion of the upper extremities in running has been almost totally ignored. Recently, Hinrichs, Cavanagh, and Williams (1983) investigated the contributions of the arms to the total angular momentum of the body. Male recreational runners ($N = 21$) were filmed while running at 3.6 m/s. The arms were found to have a substantial effect on total body angular momentum about the z (vertical) axis but little effect about the x (transverse) or y (anteroposterior) axes. The angular momentum attributed to the arms was found to be comparable, but in the opposite direction, to the angular momentum of the body-minus-arms about the z axis. Thus, the arms served to roughly "balance" the angular momentum generated by the legs so that the total body angular momentum about the vertical axis was very small. Even though the arms are only about one third the mass of the legs, their respective mass centers are located farther from the z axis than are the mass centers of the legs, allowing the arms to "compete favorably" with the legs about this axis (Hinrichs et al., 1983).

For increases in running speed above 3.6 m/s, it might be expected that arm motion would change in relation to the changes in leg motion that are required to produce gains in stride length and/or stride rate. Lusby (1983) conducted an investigation of speed-related position-time profiles of arm motion in trained women distance runners. Eight women subjects who were experienced at running cross-country races and marathons were filmed (150 fps) at three steady-state paces: a training pace of 3.8 m/s, a middle distance racing pace of 5.5 m/s, and a maximal sprinting pace of 6.3 to 8.1 m/s ($\overline{X}$ = 6.9 m/s).

The coordinates of the shoulder, elbow, and wrist joint centers were digitized from the side-view film. The true (3-dimensional) elbow joint angle was computed by determining the extent of out-of-plane position of the upper arm and forearm in each frame based on the ratio of apparent to true length of these segments. Upper arm position with respect to a vertical line through the shoulder joint represented shoulder flexion and extension, and full elbow extension was defined as zero degrees.

The range of motion at the shoulder and elbow joints increased as running speed increased. When the two extremes of running speed were compared, it was found that maximum shoulder joint flexion and extension during the sprinting pace carried the upper arm farther in front of the vertical ($\overline{X}$ = 34°) and behind the vertical ($\overline{X}$ = -76°) than during the training pace ($\overline{X}$ = 0° and $\overline{X}$ = -56°, respectively). Likewise, an increase from training to sprinting Pace was accompanied by an increase in both maximum elbow flexion (from $\overline{X}$ = 97° to $\overline{X}$ = 111°) and extension (from $\overline{X}$ = 70° to $\overline{X}$ = 61°).

The temporal interrelationships of the shoulder and elbow joint motions during one complete stride cycle can be illustrated using an angle-angle diagram (Figure 1) in which the angles of the upper arm and elbow are plotted

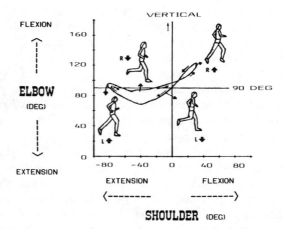

Figure 1   Angle-angle diagram for Subject 1, running at 7.12 m/s. Upper arm position was measured with respect to a vertical line through the shoulder joint, and elbow angle was measured between an extended upper arm line and the forearm so that full extension equals 0°. Points of ipsilateral (right) and contralateral (left) foot touchdown and takeoff are designated.

against one another. Figures 2a, b, and c illustrate the individual variability in arm motion for subjects 1, 2 and 3. The general shape of the plot remained quite similar within each subject across the three running speeds and depicted the increase in range of motion at faster running speeds. However, the absolute range of motion at the shoulder and elbow joints differed considerably among the subjects. For example, subject 3 showed very little deviation of the elbow joint from an 80 degree position except at the most forward point in the arm-swing. In contrast, subjects 1 and 2 flexed and extended the elbow through an increasingly larger range as running speed increased.

As Miller (1978) indicated in her discussion of the future of sport bio-mechanics research, display techniques such as the angle-angle diagram should contribute to further understanding of angular kinematics of the stride cycle as they are influenced by running velocity. Additional research also is needed to compare the performance characteristics of male and female distance runners. Biomechanists indeed have "a long distance" to go—but a sound foundation on which to build—in their quantification of kinematic and kinetic aspects of running.

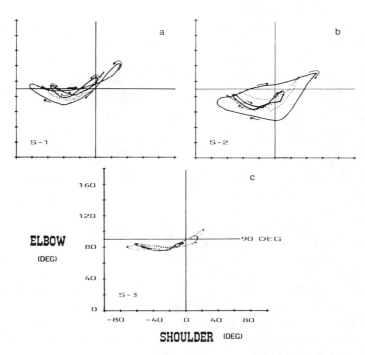

Figure 2a, b, and c Angle-angle diagrams for Subjects 1, 2, and 3. The smallest plot (solid line) on each graph represents arm motion in the training pace, the largest plot (solid line) depicts arm motion at the sprinting pace, and the intermediate plot (dotted line) reflects arm motion at the racing pace. Refer to Figure 1 for an explanation of these diagrams.

References

Dillman, C.J. (1975). Kinematic analyses of running. In J.H. Wilmore & J.F. Keogh (Eds.), *Exercise and Sport Sciences Reviews*, (3, 193-218), New York: Academic Press.

Hinrichs, R.N., Cavanagh, P.R., & Williams, K.R. (1983). Upper extremity contributions to angular momentum in running. In H. Matsui & K. Kobayashi (Eds.), *Biomechanics VIII-B*, (pp. 641-647). Champaign: Human Kinetics Publishers.

Latshaw, R.F., Kantner, T.R., Kalenak, A., Baum, S., & Corcoran, J.J. (1981). A pelvic stress fracture in a female jogger: A case report. *The American Journal of Sports Medicine*, 9(1), 54-56.

Luhtanen, P., & Komi, P.V. (1978). Mechanical factors influencing running speed. In E. Asmussen & K. Jorgensen (Eds.), *Biomechanics VI-B* (pp. 23-29). Baltimore: University Park Press.

Lusby, L.A. (1983). *Speed-related position-time profiles of arm motion in trained women distance runners.* Unpublished master's thesis. University of Arizona, Tucson.

Miller, D.I. (1978). Biomechanics of running—what should the future hold? *Canadian Journal of Applied Sport Sciences*, 3, 229-236.

Nelson, R.C., Brooks, C.M., & Pike, N.L. (1977). Biomechanical comparison of male and female distance runners. In P. Milvy (Ed.), *The marathon. Physiological, medical, epidemiological, and psychological studies* (pp. 793-807). Annals of the New York Academy of Sciences, 301. New York: The New York Academy of Sciences.

Ozburn, M.S., & Nichols, J.W. (1981). Pubic ramus and adductor insertion stress fractures in female basic trainees. *Military Medicine*, 146(5), 332-334.

Pavlov, H., Nelson, T.L., Warren, R.F., Torg, J.S., & Burstein, A.J. (1982). Stress fractures of the pubic ramus. *The Journal of Bone and Joint Surgery*, 64-A(7), 1020-1025.

Prescott, L. (1983). Pelvic stress fractures more common in women. *The Physician and Sportsmedicine*, 11(5), 25-26.

Saito, M., Kobayashi, K., Miyashita, M., & Hoshikawa, T. (1974). Temporal patterns in running. In R.C. Nelson & C.A. Morehouse (Eds.), *Biomechanics IV* (pp. 106-111). Baltimore: University Park Press.

Tehranzadeh, J., Kurth, L.A., Elyaderani, M.K., & Bowers, K.D. (1982). Combined pelvic stress fracture and avulsion of the adductor longus in a middle-distance runner: A case report. *The American Journal of Sports Medicine*, 10(2), 108-111.

5 Nutrition for the Female Distance Runner

Emily M. Haymes

Florida State University

Running is one of our most expensive sports as far as energy is concerned. A runner weighing 65 kg expends approximately 100 kcal per mile (Howley & Glover, 1974). Distance runners who run 10 miles per day need an additional 15 kcal per kg of weight (1.5 kcal/kg/mile) in their diets to balance the caloric expenditure. One question frequently asked is whether the additional calories should come mostly from carbohydrates or from a balanced mixture of carbohydrates, fats, and proteins. Early work by Christensen and Hansen (1939) reported that endurance was greater when subjects consumed a diet high in carbohydrate (> 80%) than with a normal mixed diet or a diet high in fat and protein. Thus, the concept of carbohydrate loading before exercise was born.

Carbohydrate Loading

Carbohydrates are the preferred energy source when the exercise intensity is heavy (70% $\dot{V}O_2$max and above). Most of the energy is derived from glycogen stored in the muscles. However, during prolonged heavy exercise blood glucose must also be used by the muscles. The sources of the blood glucose are glycogen stores in the liver and gluconeogenesis (glucose formed from lactic acid, pyruvic acid, amino acids, and glycerol). During prolonged light to moderate exercise, fats are a major source of energy thus sparing the need for large quantities of carbohydrate.

Unlike fat, the total amount of carbohydrate stored by the body is limited. The liver normally stores about 90 g of glycogen, and the muscle glycogen content is about 300 g after a mixed diet (Saltin, 1978). Muscle glycogen content can be doubled by first depleting the glycogen stores through strenuous exercise and then consuming a diet low in carbohydrate for three days (Bergstrom, Hermansen, Hultman, & Saltin, 1967). Similar increases in liver glycogen content have been observed following the same dietary regimen (Hultman, 1978). Unfortunately, there are several disadvantages in using this procedure. During the three days of low carbohydrate intake the person may experience hypoglycemia and may not be able to train properly. The high muscle glycogen levels were achieved by subjects who did not exercise during the three days of high carbohydrate intake. Many athletes may not be able to give up a full week of training before an event to achieve elevated muscle glycogen levels. The high (90%) and low (10%) carbohydrate diets are not balanced nutritionally and not recommended for prolonged use. According to Saltin (1978), elevated glycogen stores are not achieved with frequent use of this procedure unless separated by several weeks of a mixed diet.

It is possible to increase muscle glycogen stores without resorting to the low carbohydrate-high fats diets used by the Swedes. The key to increased muscle glycogen storage is the exercise bout that depletes the glycogen stores. Increased glycogen synthesis is observed only in muscles that have first been depleted (Bergstrom & Hultman, 1966). Using an exercise depletion-taper sequence, Sherman, Costill, Fink, and Miller (1981) compared the effects on muscle glycogen content of three days each of low (15%) and high (70%) carbohydrate diets with three days of a mixed diet (50% carbohydrate) followed by three days of high carbohydrate. Both dietary procedures significantly increased muscle glycogen to approximately 200 mmoles glucose units per kg of wet muscle. When the mixed diet was consumed for six days following depletion, muscle glycogen levels were significantly lower than after the high carbohydrate diets.

While it is well established that the depletion-carbohydrate loading procedure increases muscle glycogen content, it also increases the rate at which carbohydrates are used during exercise. Sherman et al. (1981) found that muscle glycogen stores were used at a faster rate during a 20.9 km run after carbohydrate loading than after a mixed diet. The question for the athlete in endurance events is whether performance is improved by carbohydrate loading. Performance does not appear to be improved in distance runs that are 20.9 km or less by carbohydrate loading (Costill, Sherman, Fink, Maresh, Witten, & Miller, 1981; Sherman et al., 1981). On the other hand, better performances were observed in a 30-km race after carbohydrate loading than after a mixed diet (Karlsson & Saltin, 1971). Although the initial speed was the same for both diets, the runners were able to maintain a faster pace during the latter half of the race after carbohydrate loading. Apparently, carbohydrate loading allows the runner to maintain the exercise intensity (speed) for a longer time during the run. When the glycogen stores are depleted, the exercise intensity must be reduced for fat to be used. Following a mixed diet, muscle glycogen levels in the vastus lateralis are depleted in approximately 90 min of cycling at 77% $\dot{V}O_2$max (Hermansen, Hultman, & Saltin, 1967). In other words, events lasting less than 90 min are not as likely to be helped by carbohydrate loading as those lasting more than 90 min.

Runners should maintain an elevated carbohydrate intake during training. Daily runs of 16.1 km result in a progressive depletion of the glycogen stores when the runners consume a mixed diet containing 40% to 50% of the calories as carbohydrate (Costill, Bowers, Branam, & Sparks, 1971). By increasing the carbohydrate to 70% of the calories (525 g), the amount of glycogen stored in the muscle is more than doubled 24 hr after exercise compared with a 50% carbohydrate diet (Costill et al., 1981). The form of the carbohydrates eaten also appears to be important. Although no differences in muscle glycogen content were observed after 24 hr, consumption of complex carbohydrates (starches) produced significantly higher glycogen levels after 48 hr than eating simple sugars (Costill et al., 1981).

While meals high in carbohydrate are beneficial in restoring glycogen levels following exercise, they may have a detrimental effect if they are eaten 30 min to 2 hr before an event. Ingestion of 75 g glucose 30 min before exercise significantly reduced the length of time subjects could cycle at 80% $\dot{V}O_2$max compared with trials following the ingestion of water or a liquid meal containing carbohydrate, fat, and protein (Foster, Costill, & Fink, 1979). Ingesting glucose before exercise elevates the blood glucose level and stimulates an insulin response. Once exercise begins, blood glucose levels fall rapidly and have been reported to reach hypoglycemic levels (Costill, Coyle, Dalsky, Evans, Fink, & Hoopes, 1977). Presumably, the decrease in blood glucose is a result of increased binding of insulin to muscle receptor sites, which accelerates the uptake of glucose (Bonen, Malcolm, Kilgour, MacIntyre, & Belcastro, 1981). If glucose ingestion is delayed until after exercise begins, there is no increase in insulin, and blood glucose levels are maintained during exercise.

Men Versus Women

There has been some speculation that women might be more efficient in using fat during exercise because they have a higher percent body fat than men. Ullyot (1974) suggested that women might perform better at ultramarathon distances because they are better able to use fat and are less dependent on carbohydrate as an energy source. However, studies to date have lent little support to this hypothesis. Fat mobilization and utilization during exercise have been found to be similar in men and women (Costill, Fink, Getchell, Ivy, & Witzmann, 1979; Powers, Riley, & Howley, 1980). Costill et al. (1979) found that male distance runners have a greater potential for using fat than female runners by measuring in vitro the ability of muscle tissue to oxidize fatty acids.

Ketogenic Diets and Performance

Recently it has been suggested that adapting to a ketogenic diet might be beneficial in endurance events (Phinney, Bistrian, Evans, Gervino, & Blackburn, 1983). Ketogenic diets are low in carbohydrate and high in fat and are popular for losing body weight rapidly. By reducing the amount of carbohydrate available for glycogen synthesis, the liver is forced to use other substrates to maintain blood glucose levels. Amino acids, lactic acid, and glycerol are converted to glucose through gluconeogenesis. After several days of a low carbohydrate diet, less glucose is removed from the blood as the tissues begin to use ketone bodies for energy (Hultman, 1978). The liver increases its production of acetoacetate and β-hydroxy-butyrate (ketogenesis) after a few days of a low carbohydrate diet.

Endurance has been found to be drastically reduced after several days of a low carbohydrate diet (Christensen & Hansen, 1939; Galbo, Holst, & Christensen, 1979; Pruett, 1970). However, recent work by Phinney et al. (1983) suggests that there is no reduction in endurance if subjects are allowed four weeks of adaptation to the diet. The subjects (trained cyclists) exercised at 62% to 64% of $\dot{V}O_2$max on a cycle ergometer to exhaustion. After 4 weeks of a low (2%) carbohydrate diet, the subjects were able to complete the same amount of work while utilizing primarily fats as the energy source.

Most distance runners work at a higher %$\dot{V}O_2$max during training and races. When subjects exercise at 85% $\dot{V}O_2$max, time to exhaustion is still reduced after three weeks of a low (2% to 6%) carbohydrate diet (Cooney, 1983). While ketogenic diets may not have a negative effect on light to moderate exercise, it would appear that heavy exercise is adversely affected by a low carbohydrate intake for at least three weeks.

Use of Protein for Energy

For a long time it was believed that protein metabolism was not a significant source of energy during exercise because of the low nitrogen excretion in the urine after exercise. However, several recent studies have focused attention on the elevated urea nitrogen content of the sweat (Cerny, 1975, Dohm, Williams,Kasperek, & van Rij, 1982; Lemon & Mullin, 1980). Dohm et al. (1982) found a significantly increased urea excretion after a 16.1-km run, which suggested an increase in protein catabolism during and after exercise. Larger amounts of urea appear in the sweat and serum after carbohydrate depletion than after carbohydrate loading (Konopka & Haymes, 1983; Lemon & Mullin, 1980). Because most of the nitrogen from proteins is converted to urea, it has been suggested that increased urea levels are due to an increase in protein catabolism. When the glycogen stores are depleted, protein catabolism could supply amino acids for the liver to convert to glucose.

Alanine is thought to be the primary amino acid converted to glucose by the liver during moderate exercise (Felig & Wahren, 1971). Other amino acids, particularly the branched-chain amino acids, can be converted to alanine in the tissues through transamination. Significantly reduced serum levels of alanine and the branch-chain amino acids (leucine, isoleucine, and valine) have been observed following a 70-km ski race (Refsum, Gjessing, & Stromme, 1979) and a 100-km run (Decombaz, Reinhardt, Anantharaman, von Glutz, & Poortmans, 1979). Reduced alanine levels could mean reduced availability of substrate for gluconeogenesis during prolonged heavy exercise or the use of another amino acid (glutamate/glutamine) as the major source of glucose (Refsum et al., 1979).

The source of the amino acids catabolized during exercise has not been conclusively identified. If muscle fibers are destroyed during or after exercise, 3-methylhistidine excretion should increase. Dohm et al. (1982) reported a significant increase in 3-methylhistidine excretion following a 16.1-km run; however, no significant increase in 3-methylhistidine excretion was seen following a 100-km run (Decombaz et al., 1979). Another possible source would be the amino acid pool in the liver. If protein synthesis decreases during exercise, these amino acids would be available for use by the muscle and liver as energy sources. Because the rate at which leucine is catabolized increases while the rate at which leucine is incorporated into protein decreases during exercise, it has been suggested that protein synthesis decreases during prolonged moderate exercise (Evans, Fisher, Hoerr, & Young, 1983).

Estimates of the amount of energy derived from protein during moderate exercise range from 4% (Lemon & Mullin, 1979) to 18% (Dohm et al., 1982) of the calories expended. For a 60-kg runner who runs 10 miles a day (approximately 1,000 kcal) this would require an additional 10 to 45 g of protein ([0.04 × 1,000 kcal]/4 kcal/g of protein = 10 g of protein). The Recommended Dietary Allowance (RDA) for protein is 0.8 g/kg weight for adults. If 4% of the energy is derived from protein, then the 60-kg runner would need approximately 1 g/kg ([60 kg × 0.8 g/k] + 10 g = 58 g). The need for specific essential amino acids, the branched-chain amino acids, may be even greater than estimated from the protein requirement. Evans et al. (1983) estimated that 90% of the leucine requirement was oxidized during 2 hrs of moderate exercise. Further research is needed before recommendations on a protein requirement during exercise can be made.

The Need for Iron

Iron deficiency is common among women distance runners (Clement & Asmundson, 1982; Hunding, Jordal, & Paulev, 1981; Nickerson & Tripp, 1983; Plowman & McSwegin, 1981). Until recently low iron stores were thought to be a problem exclusively for women athletes. However, evidence of iron depletion among men runners has accumulated over the past five years (see Table 1). Low or absent iron stores in the bone marrow (Ehn, Carlmark, & Hoglund, 1979; Wishnitzer, Vorst, & Berrebi, 1983) and low serum ferritin levels (Clement & Asmundson, 1982; Dufaux, Hoederath, Streitberger, Hollmann, & Assmann, 1981) have been reported for men distance runners. The cause of the low iron stores has been the subject of numerous investigators.

Table 1 Percentage of Endurance Athletes Who Were Iron Deficient

Study	Sex	Sport	% Anemic	% Iron Deficient
Clement & Asmundson	M	Runners	10.5	29 (a)
	F	Runners	0	82 (a)
Dufaux et al.	M	Runners		8 (a)
Ehn et al.	M	Runners		100 (b)
Haymes et al.	M	Skiers	0	22 (a)
	F	Skiers	0	60 (a)
Hunding et al.	M	Runners	0	13 (c)
	F	Runners	3	39 (c)
Nickerson & Tripp	F	Runners	11	50 (a)
Plowman & McSwegin	F	Runners	18.5	33 (c)
Wishnitzer et al.	M	Runners		54 (b)

Method of determining iron deficiency: (a) low serum ferritin; (b) bone marrow iron absent or only trace amount; (c) low percent transferrin saturation.

To remain in iron balance, the iron absorbed from the diet must equal the amount of iron lost by the body. Under normal circumstances, men and nonmenstruating women lose approximately 1 mg of iron a day through the urine, feces, sweat, and desquamation of cells. Women with normal menstrual cycles lose about 1.5 mg per day, the additional iron being lost in the menses. Approximately 10% of the dietary iron intake is absorbed in the small intestine and the remainder is excreted in the feces. Iron balance should be achieved by men if the iron intake is 10 mg/day. For women, the RDA has been set at 18 mg iron/day to allow for the variation in iron loss through the menses. The normal dietary iron intake is 6 mg/1,000 kcal. While adult men have little trouble meeting the RDA of 10 mg, the average dietary intakes for women range from 10 to 12 mg of iron per day (White, 1968). Thus it is not really a surprise that many women athletes are iron deficient. Under normal circumstances men have approximately 1,000 mg of iron stored in the bone marrow, liver, and spleen, while women have up to 400 mg of stored iron. If iron loss exceeds iron intake, iron is taken from the stores to produce hemoglobin, myoglobin, cytochrome c, and the enzymes containing iron.

One of the early indicators of depleted iron stores is a low serum ferritin level (Bothwell, Charlton, Cook, & Finch, 1979). Ferritin concentration below 12 ug/1 is considered a good indication that the iron stores are completely depleted. Distance runners, both men and women, have been reported to have significantly lower ferritin levels than other athletes and less physically active persons (Dufaux et al., 1981; Haymes, unpublished data). Other evidence that iron is being used at a faster rate than it is being replaced is an increase in transferrin concentration and elevated free erythrocyte porphyrin (FEP) levels. Both have been observed during training for cross-country running (Frederickson, Puhl, & Runyan, 1983) and cross-country skiing (Haymes, Puhl, & Temples, 1983). Although low iron intake is often suspected to be the cause of iron depletion in women athletes, dietary iron intake for the women distance runners was not significantly different from that of the other women. It appears more likely that distance runners lose iron at a faster rate than other athletes, since Ehn et al. (1979) found that men runners lose approximately 2 mg of iron a day.

The two most likely sources of iron loss during exercise are sweating and red blood cell destruction with hemoglobin and/or iron lost in the urine. Sweat iron concentration ranges from 0.13 to 0.4 mg/l (Paulev, Jordal, & Pedersen, 1983; Vellar, 1968). Runners who lose up to 3 l of sweat per day could be losing as much as 1 mg of iron per day in the sweat. Evidence of increased red blood cell destruction has also been observed among distance runners. Red blood cells are more fragile during the first few weeks of training, which is partly responsible for the "sports anemia" observed at the beginning of training (Puhl, Runyan, & Kruse, 1981). Low serum haptoglobin levels are also an indication of increased red blood cell destruction. Distance runners have lower serum haptoglobin levels than other athletes (Dufaux et al., 1981). When red blood cells are destroyed in the bloodstream, haptoglobin picks up the hemoglobin and is then removed by the liver. If more hemoglobin is released than can be removed by the haptoglobin, some of the hemoglobin will be removed by the kidneys and appear in the urine. Hematuria has been observed in male distance runners after a marathon (Siegel, Hennekens, Solomon, & Van Boeckel, 1979).

When the iron stores are depleted, less iron is available for hemoglobin formation and the hemoglobin concentration decreases. Because the oxygen-carrying capacity of the blood depends on the hemoglobin concentration, low hemoglobin levels are associated with a reduced maximal oxygen uptake and physical work capacity (Edgerton, Ohira, Hettiarachchi, Senewiratne, Gardner, & Barnard, 1981; Gardner, Edgerton, Senewiratne, Barnard, & Ohira, 1977; Sproule, Mitchell, & Miller, 1960). During submaximal exercise, a reduction in hemoglobin can be overcome by increasing cardiac output. Freedson (1980) found that cardiac output at a given $\dot{V}O_2$ is inversely related to the hemoglobin concentration.

Iron depletion of the tissues may have an additional effect on endurance performance. When hemoglobin concentration of iron-deficient rats was restored by transfusion, endurance did not improve and blood lactate levels were still elevated (Finch, Gollnick, Hlastala, Miller, Dillman, & Mackler, 1979). Iron deficiency was associated with a 50% reduction in the cytochrome c and cytochrome oxidase content of skeletal muscles (McLane, Fell, McKay, Winder, Brown, & Holloszy, 1981). McLane et al. (1981) found a significant improvement in muscular endurance, cytochrome c, and cytochrome oxidase, and reduced muscle lactate following iron treatment. Iron treatment of iron-deficient humans results in lower blood lactate levels (Schoene, Escourrou, Robertson, Nilson, Parsons & Smith, 1983) and lower heart rates during exercise before a significant increase in hemoglobin occurs (Ohira, Edgerton, Gardner, Gunawardena, Senewiratne, & Ikawa, 1981).

Iron supplements have been shown to be very effective in improving the performance of anemic subjects (Gardner, Edgerton, Barnard, & Bernauer, 1975; Ohira, Edgerton, Gardner, Senewiratne, Barnard, & Simpson, 1979). The question is whether iron supplements would be beneficial for athletes in training. Recent studies have reported mixed results (see Table 2). Both Plowman and McSwegin (1981) and Hunding et al. (1981) found that distance runners increased their hemoglobin levels after iron supplementation. Schoene et al. (1983) reported increases in hemoglobin, serum ferritin, and percent iron saturation in women athletes receiving iron supplements. On the other hand, Cooter and Mowbray (1978), Haymes et al. (1983), and Pate, Maguire, and Van Wyk (1979) failed to find significant improvements in hemoglobin and serum iron levels of athletes following several months of iron treatment, although Haymes et al. found lower transferrin levels in subjects receiving iron. The improvements observed by Plowman & McSwegin, Hunding et al., Nickerson & Tripp, and Schoene et al. may have been due to the large number of iron-deficient subjects in these studies coupled with the use of fairly large iron supplements. Because little iron is excreted by the body, there is danger of iron toxicity when large iron supplements are used. It is recommended that athletes have their iron status evaluated annually and that iron supplements should be taken by persons with low serum ferritin and/or hemoglobin levels.

Table 2 Effects of Iron Supplementation During Training on Hematologic and Iron Status

Study	Sport	Amount of Iron in Supplement		Increased Hemoglobin	Increased Ferritin
Cooter & Mowbray	Basketball	18 mg	(a)	no	—
Haymes et al.	X-C Skiing	18 mg	(a)	no	no
Hunding et al.	Running	74 mg	(b)	yes	—
Nickerson & Tripp	Running	60 mg	(b)	yes	yes
Pate et al.	Variety	50 mg	(b)	no	—
Plowman & McSwegin	Running	234 mg	(b)	yes	—
Schoene et al.	Variety	270 mg	(b)	yes	yes

(a) ferrous fumarate
(b) ferrous sulfate

References

Bergstrom, J., Hermansen, L., Hultman, E., & Saltin, B. (1967). Diet, muscle glycogen and physical performance. *Acta Physiologica Scandinavica,* **71**, 140-150.

Bergstrom, J., & Hultman, E. (1966). Muscle glycogen synthesis after exercise: An enhancing factor localized to the muscle cells in man. *Nature,* **210**, 309.

Bonen, A., Malcolm, S.A., Kilgour, R.D., MacIntyre, K.P., & Belcastro, A.N. (1981). Glucose ingestion before and during intense exercise. *Journal of Applied Physiology: Respiratory, Environmental and Exercise Physiology,* **50**, 766-771.

Bothwell, T.H., Charlton, R.W., Cook J.D., & Finch, C.A. (1979). *Iron metabolism in man.* Oxford: Blackwell Scientific Publications.

Cerny, F. (1975). Protein metabolism during two hour ergometer exercise. In H. Howald & J.R. Poortmans (Eds.), *Metabolic adaptation to prolonged physical exercise* (pp. 232-237). Basel: Birkhauser Verlag.

Christensen, E.H., & Hansen, O. (1939). Arbeitsfahigkeit und ernahrung. *Skandinavian Archives of Physiology,* **81**, 160-171.

Clement, D.B., & Asmundson, R.C. (1982). Nutritional intake and hematological parameters in endurance runners. *The Physician and Sportsmedicine,* **10** (3), 37-43.

Cooney, M.M. (1983). *The effects of a low carbohydrate-ketogenic diet in trained females.* Unpublished doctoral dissertation, The Florida State University.

Cooter, G.R., & Mowbray, K. (1978). Effects of iron supplementation and activity on serum iron depletion and hemoglobin levels in female athletes. *Research Quarterly,* **49**, 114-118.

Costill, D.L., Bowers, R., Branam, G., & Sparks, K. (1971). Muscle glycogen utilization during prolonged exercise on successive days. *Journal of Applied Physiology,* **31**, 834-838.

Costill, D.L., Coyle, E., Dalsky, G., Evans, W., Fink, W., & Hoopes, D. (1977). Effects of elevated FFA and insulin on muscle glycogen usage during exercise. *Journal of Applied Physiology: Respiratory, Environmental and Exercise Physiology,* **43**, 695-699.

Costill, D.L., Fink, W.J., Getchell, L.H., Ivy, J.L., & Witzmann, F.A. (1979). Lipid metabolism in skeletal muscle of endurance-trained males and females. *Journal of Applied Physiology: Respiratory, Environmental and Exercise Physiology,* **47**, 787-791.

Costill, D.L., Sherman, W.M., Fink, W.J., Maresh, C., Witten, M., & Miller, J.M. (1981). The role of dietary carbohydrates in muscle glycogen resynthesis after strenuous running. *American Journal of Clinical Nutrition,* **34**, 1831-1836.

Decombaz, J., Reinhardt, P., Anantharaman, K., von Glutz, G., & Poortmans, J.R. (1979). Biochemical changes in a 100 km run: free amino acids, urea, and creatinine. *European Journal of Applied Physiology, 41*, 61-72.

Dohm, G.L., Williams, R.T., Kasperek, G.J., & van Rij, A.M. (1982). Increased excretion of urea and N-methylhistidine by rats and humans after a bout of exercise. *Journal of Applied Physiology: Respiratory, Environmental, and Exercise Physiology, 52*, 27-33.

Dufaux, B., Hoederath, A., Streitberger, I., Hollman, W., & Assmann, G. (1981). Serum ferritin, transferrin, haptoglobin, and iron in middle- and long-distance runners, elite rowers, and professional racing cyclists. *International Journal of Sports Medicine, 2*, 43-46.

Edgerton, V.R., Ohira, Y., Hettiarachchi, J., Senewiratne, B., Gardner, G.W., & Barnard, R.J. (1981). Elevation of hemoglobin and work tolerance in iron deficient subjects. *Journal of Nutrition Science and Vitaminology, 27*, 77-86.

Ehn, L., Carlmark, B., & Hoglund, S. (1979). Iron status in athletes involved in intense physical activity. *Medicine and Science in Sports and Exercise, 12*, 61-64.

Evans, W.J., Fisher, E.C., Hoerr, R.A., & Young, V.R. (1983). Protein metabolism and endurance exercise. *The Physician and Sportsmedicine, 11* (7): 63-72.

Felig, P., & Wahren, J. (1971). Amino acid metabolism in exercising man. *Journal of Clinical Investigation, 50*, 2703-2714.

Finch, C.A., Gollnick, P.D., Hlastala, M.P., Miller, L.R., Dillman, E., & Mackler, B. (1979). Lactic acidosis as a result of iron deficiency. *Journal of Clinical Investigation, 64*, 129-137.

Foster, C., Costill, D.L., & Fink, W.J. (1979). Effects of preexercise feedings on endurance performance. *Medicine and Science in Sports, 11*, 1-5.

Frederickson, L.A., Puhl, J.L., & Runyan, W.S. (1983). Effects of training on indices of iron status of young female cross-country runners. *Medicine and Science in Sports and Exercise, 15*, 271-276.

Freedson, P.S. (1981). The influence of hemoglobin concentration on exercise cardiac output. *International Journal of Sports Medicine, 2*, 81-86.

Galbo, H., Holst, J.J., & Christensen, N.J. (1979). The effect of different diets and insulin on the hormonal response to prolonged exercise. *Acta Physiologica Scandinavica, 107*, 19-32.

Gardner, G.W., Edgerton, V.R., Barnard, R.J. & Bernauer, E.M. (1975). Cardiorespiratory, hematological and physical performance responses of anemic subjects to iron treatment. *American Journal of Clinical Nutrition, 28*, 982-988.

Gardner, G.W., Edgerton, V.R., Senewiratne, B., Barnard, R.J., & Ohira, Y. (1977). Physical work capacity and metabolic stress in subjects with iron deficiency anemia. *American Journal of Clinical Nutrition, 30*, 910-917.

Haymes, E.M., Puhl, J.L., & Temples, T.E. (1983). Training for cross-country skiing and iron status. *Medicine and Science in Sports and Exercise,* **14**, 133.

Hermansen, L., Hultman, E., & Saltin, B. (1967). Muscle glycogen during prolonged severe exercise. *Acta Physiologica Scandinavica,* **71**, 129-139.

Howley, E.T., & Glover, M.E. (1974). The caloric costs of running and walking one mile for men and women. *Medicine and Science in Sports,* **6**, 235-237.

Hultman, E. (1978). Liver as a glucose supplying source during rest and exercise, with special reference to diet. In J. Parizkova & V.A. Rogozkin (Eds.), *Nutrition, Physical Fitness, and Health* (pp. 9-30). Baltimore: University Park Press.

Hunding, A., Jordal, R., & Paulev, P.E. (1981). Runner's anemia and iron deficiency. *Acta Physiologica Scandinavica,* **209**, 315-318.

Karlsson, J., & Saltin, B. (1971). Diet, muscle glycogen, and endurance performance. *Journal of Applied Physiology,* **31**: 203-206.

Konopka, B.J., & Haymes, E.M. (1983). Effect of sweat collection methods on protein contribution. *Medicine and Science in Sports and Exercise,* **15**, 99.

Lemon, P.W.R., & Mullin, J.P. (1980). Effect of initial muscle glycogen levels on protein catabolism during exercise. *Journal of Applied Physiology: Respiratory, Environmental and Exercise Physiology,* **48**, 624-629.

McLane, J.A., Fell, R.D., McKay, R.H., Winder, W.W., Brown, E.B., & Holloszy, J.O. (1981). Physiological and biochemical effects of iron deficiency on rat skeletal muscle. *American Journal of Physiology,* **241**, C47-C54.

Nickerson, H.J., & Tripp, A.D. (1983). Iron deficiency in adolescent cross-country runners. *The Physician and Sportsmedicine,* **11** (6), 60-66.

Ohira, Y., Edgerton, V.R., Gardner, G.W., Gunawardena, K.A., Senewiratne, B., & Ikawa, S. (1981). Work capacity after iron treatment as a function of hemoglobin and iron deficiency. *Journal of Nutrition Science and Vitaminology,* **27**, 87-96.

Ohira, Y., Edgerton, V.R., Gardner, G.W., Senewiratne, B., Barnard, R.J., & Simpson, D.R. (1979). Work capacity, heart rate and blood lactate responses to iron treatment. *British Journal of Haematology,* **41**, 365-372.

Pate, R.R., Maguire, M., & Van Wyk, J. (1979). Dietary iron supplementation in women athletes. *The Physician and Sportsmedicine,* **7** (9), 81-88

Paulev, P.E., Jordal, R., & Pedersen, N.S. (1983). Dermal excretion of iron in intensely training athletes. *Clinica Chimica Acta,* **127**, 19-27.

Phinney, S.D., Bistrian, B.R., Evans, W.J., Gervino, E., & Blackburn, G.L. (1983). The human metabolic response to chronic ketosis without caloric restriction: preservation of submaximal exercise capability with reduced carbohydrate oxidation. *Metabolism,* **32**, 769-776.

Plowman, S.A., & McSwegin, P.C. (1981). The effects of iron supplemen-
    tation on female cross-country runners. *Journal of Sports Medicine, 21*,
    407-416.
Powers, S.K., Riley, W., & Howley, E.T. (1980). Comparison of fat
    metabolism between trained men and women during prolonged aerobic
    work. *Research Quarterly for Exercise and Sport, 51*, 427-431.
Pruett, E.D.R. (1970). Glucose and insulin during prolonged work stress in
    men living on different diets. *Journal of Applied Physiology, 28*, 199-208.
Puhl, J.L., Runyan, W.S., & Kruse, S.J. (1981). Erythrocyte changes during
    training in high school women cross-country runners. *Research Quarterly
    for Exercise and Sport, 52*, 484-494.
Refsum, H.E., Gjessing, L.R., Stromme, S.B., (1979). Changes in plasma
    amino acid distribution and urine amino acids excretion during prolonged
    heavy exercise. *Scandinavian Journal of Clinical Laboratory Investigation,
    39*, 407-413.
Saltin, B. (1978). Fluid, electrolyte, and energy losses and their replenishment
    in prolonged exercise. In J. Parizkova & V.A. Rogozkin (Eds.), *Nutrition,
    Physical Fitness, and Health* (pp. 76-97). Baltimore: University Park
    Press.
Schoene, R.B., Escourrou, P., Robertson, H.T., Nilson, K.L., Parsons, J.R.,
    & Smith, N.J. (1983). Iron repletion decreases maximal exercise lactate
    concentrations in female athletes with minimal iron-deficiency anemia.
    Journal of Laboratory Clinical Medicine, 102, 306-312.
Sherman, W.M., Costill, D.L., Fink, W.J., & Miller, J.M. (1981). Effect
    of exercise-diet manipulation on muscle glycogen and its subsequent
    utilization during performance. *International Journal of Sports Medicine,
    2*, 114-118.
Siegel, A.J., Hennekens, C.H., Solomon, H.S., & Van Boeckel, B. (1979).
    Exercise-related hematuria: Findings in a group of marathon runners.
    Journal of the American Medical Assocation, 241, 391-392.
Sproule, B.J., Mitchell, J.H., & Miller, W.F. (1960). Cardiopulmonary
    physiological responses to heavy exercise in patients with anemia. *Journal
    of Clinical Investigation, 39*, 378-388.
Ullyot, J. (1974). Women's secret weapon: Fat. *Runner's World, 9* (12), 22-23.
Vellar, O.D. (1968). Studies on the sweat losses of nutrients. I. Iron content
    of whole body sweat and its association with other sweat constituents,
    serum iron levels, hematological indices, body surface area, and sweat
    rate. *Scandinavian Journal of Clinical Laboratory Investigation, 21*,
    157-167.
White, H.S. (1968). Iron nutriture of girls and women—a review. *Journal
    of the American Dietetic Association, 53*, 563-569.
Wishnitzer, R., Vorst, E., & Berrebi, A. (1983). Bone marrow iron depression
    in competitive distance runners. *International Journal of Sports Medicine,
    4*, 24-30.

6

Effects of Marathon Running on Blood Chemistry Profiles

Christine L. Wells, Joel R. Stern, Lillian M. Hecht

Arizona State University

Long-distance running provides a significant stress on the human body. Even the exceptionally well-trained runner experiences considerable thermal, metabolic, and circulatory stress both during the course of endurance training and during a competitive event. Many (if not all) of these changes, responses, and adaptations are reflected in a runner's blood chemistry profile. Because the effects of marathon running on blood chemistry profiles are so complicated and involve so many variables, this paper is divided into six parts to present as logical a progression as possible. This division of parameters is arbitrary; readers may differ with the placement of a particular parameter.

The first part deals with hematological changes that indicate fluid compartment shifts. The second part includes red and white blood cell changes, and the third part is limited to serum protein and electrolyte changes. The fourth section discusses substances involved with carbohydrate (CHO) and lipid metabolism. Much has been written on this topic, which has ramifications for substrate utilization, weight control and obesity, and heart and circulatory disease. We chose not to develop these topics because they have been discussed elsewhere. The fifth part deals with substances related to metabolic turnover and/or cell injury; and the sixth part deals with changes in serum enzymes. A discussion of specific results will be included within each section to avoid an unmanageable general discussion. We have attempted to compare the responses of female runners with male runners, but because few studies have been completed with women long-distance runners, this aspect of the paper is not as well developed as would be desirable.

The authors are gratefully indebted to Dr. Gary S. Krahenbuhl for his assistance with statistical analyses. We are also greatly appreciative of the extraordinary efforts of the subjects. For technical assistance we wish to thank Jean Olson, R.N.; Bonnie Meyers, R.N.; Susan Grambly, R.N.; Jack Levine, Technicon Corporation; Jerry Hill, National Health Laboratories; and Edward Smith, M.D.

This study was supported by an Arizona State University faculty grant-in-aid; the Dean's Research Fund, Arizona State University; and Technicon Corporation (Terrytown, N.Y.).

Methods and Procedures

Six male and four female runners competing in the Fiesta Bowl Marathon (Scottsdale, AZ), took part in the study. Some descriptive characteristics of the subjects are presented in Table 1. These subjects have been described extensively in a previous paper (Wells, Hecht, & Krahenbuhl, 1981). Basically, these runners can be classified as good (i.e., better than average, but not elite) performers.

Table 1 Descriptive Variables of the Subjects

Gender	Age (years)	Height (cm)	Weight (kg)	Surface area (m²)	LBM (kg)	$\dot{V}O_2$max (ml•kg^{-1}•min^{-1})
Men	30.8	179.5[a]	70.1[a]	1.87[a]	64.7[a]	58.41
n = 6	±8.7	±5.4	±5.8	±0.69	±5.6	±5.00
Women	28.5	166.6[a]	52.0[a]	1.56[a]	46.1[a]	59.20
n = 4	±5.3	±5.5	±8.2	±0.13	±7.7	±7.14

[a]$p < .001$, men larger than women
Values are means ± SD

At the 8 a.m. start of the race, the ambient temperature was 10.6° C with 67% relative humidity. At the finish of the race, these measurements were 15° C and 48%. A strong wind (31.5 kmh) lowered the equivalent still-air temperature to 1° C when the race began. The wind lessened at 11 a.m., and the equivalent still-air temperature rose to 3.9° C. It was completely cloudy. The course was relatively flat and the road surface was macadam.

All the runners consumed water and/or a glucose-electrolyte solution (ERG) during competition. No attempt was made to control or measure the liquids consumed, but the runners were urged to drink as they usually did. After the race the subjects were instructed to eat and drink as they usually would following such a race.

Blood samples taken immediately before a marathon may not represent a true resting state because of anxiety and special dietary preparations such as carbohydrate loading (Maron, Horvath, & Wilkerson, 1977). Therefore, "control" blood samples were obtained one week before the race. Subjects rested in a sitting position for 30 minutes before the control samples were collected. To account for possible diurnal variation, the samples were collected at the time that corresponded to the subjects' expected finishing times. A medical history, various body measurements, and informed consent were also obtained at this time.

The first (IMM) postrace blood sample was obtained as soon as possible after the runner finished; in every case this was within 5 min. The second postrace specimen (4 H) was collected 4 hr, the third (8 H) 8 hr, and the fourth sample (24 H) 24 hr after the race. All blood samples (15 ml) were obtained from an antecubital vein without stasis using vacutainer tubes. The subjects were in a seated position. The blood used for biochemical analysis was centrifuged for 15 min and the separated serum kept at 4.5° C until processing. A Coulter Counter (Model S) was used to measure hemoglobin (Hb), hematocrit (HCT), mean cell volume (MCV), red blood cell count (RBC), white blood cell count (WBC), mean corpuscular hemoglobin (MCH), and mean corpuscular hemoglobin concentration (MCHC). Differential counts for polymorphonuclear cells (PMN) and lymphocytes (LYMPH) were also performed. Osmotic pressure measurements (freezing point depression, Advanced Osmometer, model 3L) were obtained on the anticoagulated plasma that remained after hematologic measurements were completed. A Technicon Auto-Analyzer (SMAC) was used to determine serum sodium (Na), potassium (K), chloride (C1), total protein (TP), albumin, globulin, glucose, triacylglycerol, cholesterol, blood urea nitrogen (BUN), uric acid (Urate), creatinine, total bilirubin, phosphate, and the serum enzymes lactate dehydrogenase (LDH), alkaline phosphatase (Alk Phosp), and asparate and alanine aminotransferases (ASAT and ALAT) (previously designated glutamate oxaloacetate and glutamate pyruate transaminases, or SGOT and SGPT, respectively).

Plasma volume changes (ΔPV) were calculated from Hb and HCT, corrected for trapped plasma, by the method of Dill and Costill (1974). In this way, each sample was compared with the previous sample. Since concentrations of measured values are what the body's cells actually respond to, and corrected values show the effect of plasma volume changes on these concentrations, both values will be presented.

Statistical analysis included examination for differences among sample means (Control, IMM, 4 H, 8 H, 24 H) via one-way ANOVA with repeated measures. Post-hoc analyses of significant differences among repeated measures were performed using the conservative Scheffe multiple comparison technique if F was significant at the $p < .05$ level (Winer, 1971).

Results and Discussion

Fluid compartment shifts

Figure 1 (top) illustrates the changes in Hb and HCT throughout the experimental period. Note that the women's responses were less severe than

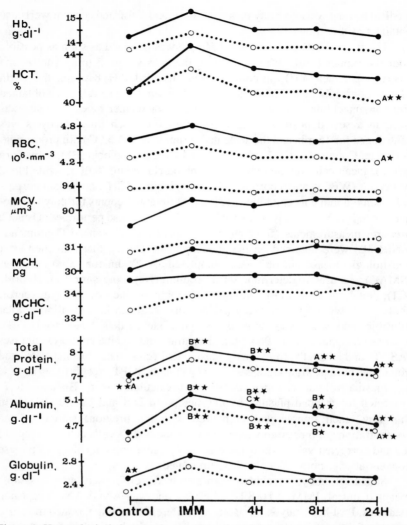

Figure 1. Hematological changes observed in male and female marathon runners. IMM, immediate postrace sample; 4H, 4 hr postrace sample; 8H, 8 hr postrace sample; 24H, 24 hr postrace sample; RCB, red blood cell count; MCV, mean corpuscular volume; MCH, mean corpuscular hemoglobin; MCHC, mean corpuscular hemoglobin concentration. Closed circles, males; open circles, females. A <IMM; B >CONTROL; C >24H; ★ p.<.05; ★★p.<.01. (Wells, Stern, & Hecht, 1982, p. 44.)

the men's. Hemoconcentration was evident immediately following the race but was essentially corrected by 24 hr.

Table 2 presents percentage changes (%Δ) in blood volume (BV), red blood cell volume (RCV), and plasma volume (PV) as calculated from Hb

Table 2 Percentage Changes in Volumes of Blood, Red Cells and Plasma Following A Marathon Race[1]

Time	Gender	% BV	% RCV	% PV
CONTROL IMM	Men	−7.2	+1.4	−12.8
	Women	−5.0	−0.8	−7.7
IMM 4 H	Men	+5.5	−0.6	+10.2
	Women	+4.4	−0.7	+7.9
4 H 8 H	Men	0.0	+0.3	−0.2
	Women	0.0	+0.5	−0.3
8 H 24 H	Men	+2.1	+1.1	+2.8
	Women	+1.5	−1.1	+3.2

BV, blood volume; RBC, red cell volume; PV, plasma volume
[1]Calculations according to Dill & Costill (1974)

and HCT values. Since RCV remained essentially unchanged, changes in BV were primarily the result of changes in PV. Immediately upon completion of the race, PV was decreased 7.7% in the women and 12.8% in the men. Similar values have been reported by others. For example, our calculations from the data of Wilkerson, Gutin, and Horvath (1977) following treadmill running at 30% to 90% $\dot{V}O_2$max in men revealed PV reductions ranging from 11% to 18%. Immediately following a marathon (ambient temperature 20.6° C), Kolka, Stephenson, Witten, Fee, and Wilkerson (1978) reported that calculated PV decreased by 10.75%, and RCV decreased by 3.12% in three males. PV reductions of 5.4%, 13.2%, and 27.4% following a warm-weather marathon (15.5 to 24.4° C WBGT) were reported in three male finishers by Myhre, Hartung, and Tucker (1982). The initial decrease in PV was expected, because Costill and Fink (1974) reported decreases of 16% to 18% in PV following a 2-hour period of treadmill exercise to 4% dehydration.

Hemodilution occurred after the race, with most of the fluid shift taking place in the plasma compartment. PV had essentially returned to control values in both groups by the 4 H specimen, with only minor changes occurring at the 8 H and 24 H mark (Wells, Stern, & Hecht, 1982). Maron et al. (1977), using the same method for calculating changes in PV, estimated that PV remained elevated for two days following a marathon. Kolka et al. (1978) reported that hemodilution persisted for eight days after a race. These latter two studies had occurred under considerably warmer circumstances. A similar pattern of hemoconcentration followed by hemodilution was reported by Dickson, Dickinson, and Noakes (1982) after a 56-km race.

RBC and WBC parameters

Figure 1 (middle portion) illustrates the changes observed in RBC, MCV, MCH, and MCHC. The only statistically significant difference was that the women's 24 H RBC value was less than the IMM post-race RBC value (p < .05). Dickson et al. (1982) reported similar changes in RBC and MCV following a 56-km race.

Figure 2 rather dramatically illustrates the leukocytosis we observed following the marathon. WBCs were markedly elevated in both males and females after the race with a nearly complete recovery by 24 hours. The increase in WBC count was the result of an increase in polymorphonuclear cells; there were no changes in lymphocytes. Leukocytosis has been observed previously following a marathon (Wilkerson, Kolka, & Stephenson, 1979; Krebs, Scully, & Zinkgraf, 1983), and a 24-hour relay race (Williams & Ward, 1977). PMNs were significantly elevated in this latter study, but lymphocytes, monocytes, eosinophils, and basophils were not. As reported in a previous paper (Wells et al., 1982), this leukocytosis may result from two processes. First, Robbins and Angell (1976) describe "margination" as a tendency for WBCs to congregate along blood vessel walls outside the axial stream of blood flow. When blood is collected in the usual resting state these marginated cells remain in the vascular system and are not counted. The increased blood flow due to exercise may wash these cells from blood vessel walls and cause an apparent increase in WBC count, although the actual number of intravascular WBCs has not changed. Wilkerson et al. (1979) suggested that this process was at least partially responsible for the marked leukocytosis they observed in male marathon runners.

A second mechanism that may contribute to the observed post-race leukocytosis is an inflammatory response to local tissue injury. In the case of marathon runners this might result from repeated impact of the feet against the ground and perhaps from severely stressed muscle tissue as well. This response would specifically cause an increase in PMN cells, which was the observed response following the race. This result suggests that the second mechanism may be chiefly responsible for the post-race leukocytosis.

Proteins and electrolyte changes

Total serum protein was significantly elevated following the race with a slow decline to the 24 H sample (see Figure 1—bottom portion). Albumin and globulin fractions followed a parallel course, although the increase in globulin was less pronounced (Wells et al., 1982). Changes in the female runners were less severe and returned to control levels somewhat more rapidly. Significant increases in total protein (Maron, Horvath, & Wilkerson, 1975), and in protein

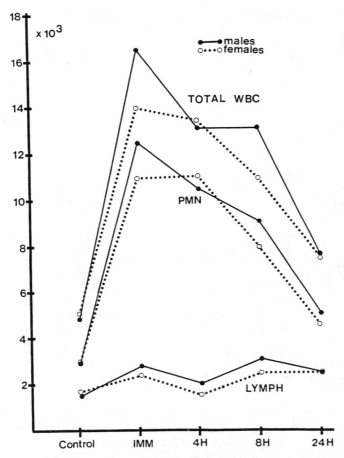

Figure 2. Leukocytosis in male and female runners following a marathon race. WBC, white blood cells; PMN, polymorphonuclear neutrophils; LYMPH, lymphocytes. Closed circles, males; open circles, females. (Wells, Stern, & Hecht, 1982, p. 45.)

and albumin (Riley, Pyke, Roberts, & England, 1975; Krebs et al., 1983) have been noted previously following marathon races in warmer environments.

Hemoconcentration may be at least a partial cause of the increases in serum proteins, but Senay (1979) offers two other possible explanations. One is that trained individuals are capable of moving protein from the interstitial spaces into the vascular compartment to form an osmotic base to combat the loss of plasma water. The other possibility is that the cold environment throughout the race stimulated the flow of lymph—with a high protein concentration—from the contracting musculature to the vascular volume.

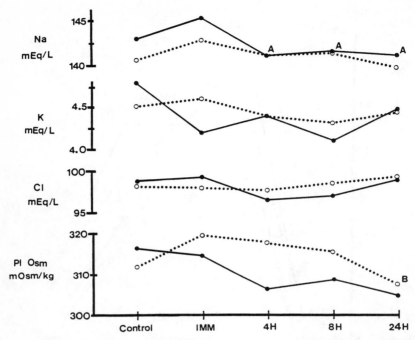

Figure 3. Serum electrolyte and plasma osmolality in male and female runners following a marathon race. Closed circles, males; open circles, females. A <IMM, p.<.05; B <IMM, p.<.01. (Wells, Stern, & Hecht, 1982, p. 46.)

Serum electrolyte concentrations (Na, K, Cl) did not change significantly from control values following the race (see Figure 3) and remained within normal ranges. The fluctuations in Na concentration seemed to parallel the course of hemoconcentration followed by hemodilution. Once again, the graphic illustration of results appears to indicate that the females had more stable values than the males for these parameters.

The literature reveals widely disparate results. For example, following marathon performance no change in serum Na was reported by Maron et al. (1977), whereas others reported increased Na (Krebs et al. 1983; Riley et al. 1975; Rose, Carroll, Lowe, Peterson, & Cooper, 1970). Increased serum K was reported by Rose et al. and Riley et al., but not by Krebs et al. Riley et al. reported an increase in serum Cl following a marathon, but Rose et al. did not. Still more confusion occurs if one examines electrolyte changes with ultramarathon performance (Dancaster & Whereat, 1971; McKechnie, Leary, & Joubert, 1967) and intermittent long-duration running (Williams & Ward, 1977). Riley et al. suggested that hemoconcentration might cause elevation of Na, K, and Cl, and that, in addition, K might be lost from cells and enter the plasma. Rose et al. proposed a similar theory. Variations in ambient temperature may be an important factor in explaining these discordant results. Senay (1979) has shown that the same exercise can yield opposite changes in hematocrit and protein when ambient temperature is changed from 20° to 30° to 40° C. Also, lymph has an electrolyte composition similar to that of plasma. The increased lymph flow from muscle at the start of exercise described by Senay (1979) might contribute water and electrolytes to plasma and blunt changes in electrolyte concentration caused by movement of water from plasma to muscle.

We did not observe significant changes in plasma osmotic pressure except that the women's 24 H value was less than the IMM value. Rose, et al. reported a small (4%) but significant rise in serum osmolality immediately following a marathon run in fair weather that corresponded with their reported increases in electrolyte concentrations.

Substances involved in Carbohydrate and Lipid Metabolism

The top portion of Figure 4 shows the progressive percentage changes in plasma volume ($\Delta\%$ PV) calculated from Hb and HCT values. The remaining three parts show changes in glucose, triacylglycerol, and cholesterol elicited by the marathon run. The solid lines represent the actual values obtained. The dotted lines represent calculated values, values adjusted for changes in plasma volume. The rise in glucose immediately after the race was not statistically significant for the women, even though the mean value exceeded the upper limit of normal, 115 mg•dl^{-1}. In the men, the measured IMM values were significantly higher than the control values ($p < .05$), but this difference was not significant when adjusted for ΔPV. Hyperglycemia is not a prominent finding after a marathon; minimal increases in blood glucose have been reported by Viru and Korge (1971) and Maron et al. (1975) and also in two runners who drank sweetened fluids during a race (Magazanik, Shapiro, Meytes, & Meytes, 1974), but these values were not corrected for hemoconcentration. Riley et al. (1975) reported no significant differences in glucose concentration throughout a 42-km run in which glucose replacement fluids were given ad lib after the first 10.5 km. Neither Krebs et al. (1983) nor Scheele, Herzog, Ritthaler, Wirth, and Weicker (1979) found a change in blood glucose after 42-km, although this latter group did report elevated glucose levels after 10- and 25-km races.

Triacylglycerol levels did not change significantly during the study; the peak at 8 H may have reflected the beer intake of several subjects and there was wide variability in this specimen. The significance of the elevated cholesterol immediately following the race ($p < .05$) disappeared when correction was made for ΔPV. Maron et al. (1975) reported a similar lack of change in triglyceride and cholesterol values, but decreased triglyceride levels have been reported by several groups following a marathon (Krebs et al., 1983; Scheele et al., 1979; Thompson, Cullinane, Henderson, & Herbert, 1980), one of which reported a significant increase in cholesterol (Krebs et al., 1983).

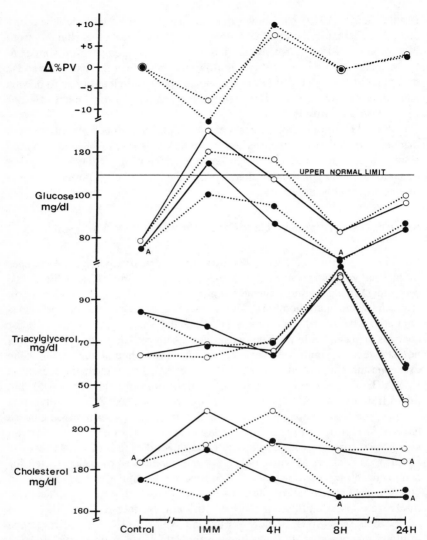

Figure 4. Percentage changes in plasma volume, blood glucose, triacylglycerol and cholesterol elicited by marathon running in men and women. Solid lines indicate measured values; dashed lines indicate values adjusted for changes in plasma volume; closed circles, males; open circles, females. A <IMM, p.<.05.

We did not examine free fatty acid (FFA) concentration or lipoprotein fractions in our subjects. However, other groups have done so and provided interesting results. For example, Scheele et al. (1979) reported that after a marathon competition the best runners had the highest increases in free fatty acids and that the longer the race (they examined runners following 10-, 25-, and 42-km races), the higher were the ß-hydroxybutyrate and acetoacetate levels. They concluded that in trained marathon runners, a shift in metabolism from glycogen to lipid oxidation occurs after covering a distance of about 25-km.

Krebs et al. (1983) examined levels of high density lipoprotein (HDL-C) and low density lipoprotein cholesterol (LDL-C) in average runners with a mean age of 37 years following a marathon in New Orleans. HDL-C levels did not change, but LDL-C levels increased significantly and remained elevated 1 to 3 weeks later. In that group of male runners, HDL-C concentration was 30%, which is between the values reported for elite and good runners, and the HDL/LDL ratio was 0.46, which is between the reported values for non-runners and good runners (Martin, Haskell, & Wood, 1977).

Substances Related to Metabolic Turnover and/or Cell Injury

High percentage changes in substances such as BUN, urate, creatinine, phosphate, and total bilirubin (see Figure 5) represent cellular constituents or products of metabolism that suggest increased metabolic turnover or cellular breakdown. BUN was not increased IMM, but was significantly elevated at 8 H in females ($p < .01$) and at 24 H in males ($p < .05$); however, all values were in the normal range. The increase in BUN agrees with findings of other investigators (Magazanik et al., 1974; Riley et al., 1975; Shapiro, Magazanik, Sohar, & Reich, 1973; Williams & Ward, 1977). In the presence of hemo-concentration and renal disease, an increase of BUN indicates increased protein catabolism caused by strenuous muscle activity in the marathon. Urate (uric acid) in females was significantly elevated above the control values in the IMM, 4 H, and 8 H specimens, but not in males; all values remained in the normal range.

The increased IMM values for creatinine were slightly blunted when adjusted for ΔPV. Considerable variability was seen in the male IMM creatinine values and statistical significance was not achieved even though the mean value was above the upper limit of normal.

Phosphate was significantly elevated in the female runners in the IMM, 4 H, and 8 H specimens, but only at 8 H in the males. In men, Riley et al. (1975) found elevated phosphate and potassium during and after a marathon and concluded that this represented a shift of ions from the intracellular to the intravascular space through increased cellular turnover.

Total bilirubin did not increase significantly after the race; others have reported elevated values following long-distance running (Gilligan, Altschule, & Katersky, 1943; Riley et al. 1975) and after intermittent long-distance running (Williams & Ward, 1977). Some (Riley et al., 1975; Williams & Ward, 1977) have suggested that an increased metabolism of hemoglobin secondary to red cell breakdown precipitated by prolonged running on hard road surfaces causes an increase in bilirubin. Earlier, Gilligan et al. (1943) had obtained evidence that hemolysis sufficient to increase bilirubin levels could not have occurred during cross-country running.

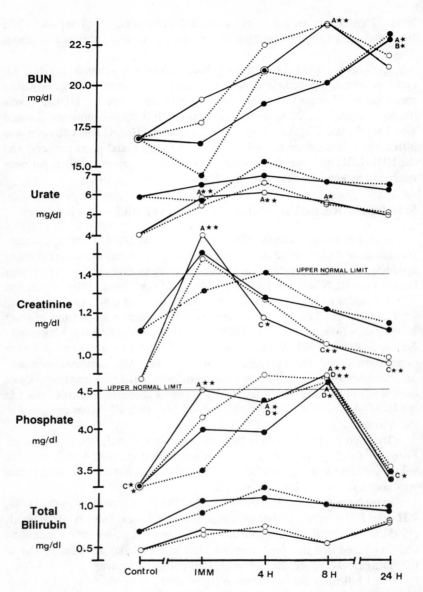

Figure 5. BUN, urate, creatinine, phosphate, and bilirubin in venous blood elicited by marathon running in men and women. Solid lines indicate measured values; dashed lines indicate values adjusted for changes in plasma volume; closed circles, males; open circles, females. A >CONTROL; B >IMM; C <IMM; D >24H; ★ p.<.05; ★★ p.<.01.

Our failure to observe statistically significant increases in urate and creatinine in the male subjects contrasts with the findings of Riley et al. (1975), Magazanik et al. (1974), and Williams and Ward (1977). Our race, however, took place with an equivalent still-air temperature of 1° to 4° C, whereas the runs of the other investigators were conducted under more moderate temperature conditions. Possibly, the cold weather on the day of our race affected the responses of these substances. Senay (1979) has reported that some physiological changes noted when exercise was performed at 20° C were reversed when the same exercise was conducted at 30° or 40° C.

It is known that blood flow to the kidneys and splanchnic bed is reduced during exercise. Castenfors (1977) reports that, although renal blood and plasma flows decrease proportionately with severity of exercise, renal regulation tends to preserve glomerular filtration, which is less markedly diminished. It seems, therefore, that the persistence of elevated BUN (24 H), urate (4 and 8 H in females) and phosphate (4 and 8 H) that we observed cannot be ascribed to impaired renal function. It seems more likely that processes responsible for these increased values—increased turnover of protein, nucleic acids, and cells—continued for these periods.

Serum Enzymes

Figure 6 illustrates the results of the serum enzymes we measured. Alkaline phosphatase (Alk Phosp), when corrected for ΔPV, did not increase after the race. Although some (Hansen, Bjerre-Knudsen, Brodthagen, Jordal, & Paulev, 1982; Riley et al. 1975) reported significant increases in Alk Phosp after long-distance running, others (Dressendorfer, Scaff, Wagner, & Gallup, 1977; Superko, Catlin, & Smith, 1979) did not. Hansen et al. (1982) credited the rise in Alk Phosp to the high bone activity in daily training athletes.

Although not statistically significant, both ASAT and ALAT increased steadily throughout the 24-hour period after the run even when adjusted for ΔPV. ASAT values markedly exceeded the upper limit of normal, and ALAT moderately exceeded them. Shapiro et al. (1972) found greatly increased ASAT and moderately increased ALAT in untrained men after a strenuous march. They concluded that the increases in these and other enzymes were most likely caused by muscle injury or increased permeability of muscle cell membranes and not by liver injury. Similar findings and conclusions have been expressed by others following marathon races (Magazanik et al., 1974; McKechnie et al., 1967). More recently, very elevated values of ASAT (Noakes and Carter, 1982) and both ASAT and ALAT (Hansen et al., 1982) have been observed and attributed to skeletal muscle cell leakage due to increased sarcolemma permeability with prolonged stress.

Control levels of LDH were at the upper limit of the normal range in our subjects. High baseline LDH levels have been reported previously in both fe-

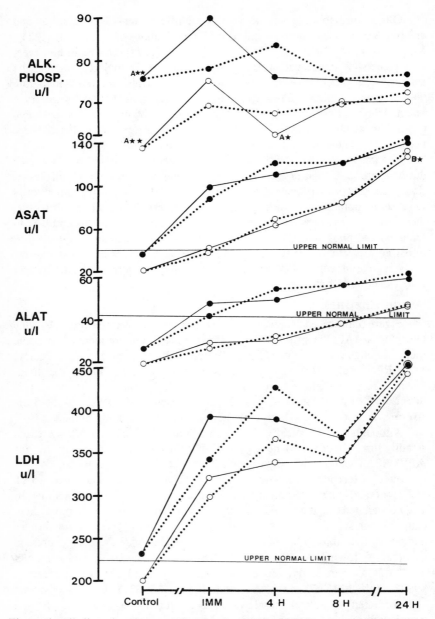

Figure 6. Alkaline phosphatase (Alk Phosp), ASAT, ALAT, and LDH elicited by marathon running in men and women. Solid lines indicate measured values; dashed lines indicate values adjusted for changes in plasma volume; closed circles, males; open circles, females. A <IMM; B >CONTROL; ★ p.<.05; ★★p.<.01.

male (Dale, Gerlach, Martin, & Alexander, 1979) and male (Martin et al., 1977) distance runners. According to Hunter and Critz (1971), resting plasma LDH activity is elevated after training. In our study, LDH increased steadily following the race, and like ASAT and ALAT, was still elevated 24 hours afterwards. Elevated LDH after a marathon has been reported previously (Dressendorfer et al., 1977; Krebs et al., 1983; Riley et al., 1975; Rose, Bousser, & Cooper, 1970). Riley et al. (1975) reported that LDH remained elevated 20 to 30 hours after a race, while Krebs et al. (1983) reported high values remained 1 to 3 weeks later.

Block, Van Rijmenant, Badjov, Van Melsem, & Vogeleer (1969) studied LDH isoenzymes for two hours following a 30-minute power test on a bicycle ergometer and concluded that the increased serum LDH level was mainly of liver and muscle origin, excluding the notion that hemolysis was responsible. Although Riley et al. (1975) were able to show that increased creatine phosphokinase (CPK) and ASAT were the results of skeletal muscle activity, they were unable to do so for LDH. LDH isoenzymes have been studied after a 10-km race (Rose, Lowe, Carroll, Wolfson, & Cooper, 1970) and following a marathon (Rose, Bousser, & Cooper, 1970). In the shorter race, only LDH-5, arising from skeletal muscle, liver, and platelets, was elevated. After the marathon, increases were noted in LDH-3, -4, and -5, but not in LDH-1 or -2. Since CPK was also significantly increased, the rise in serum enzymes was attributed mainly to skeletal muscle.

Whereas Krebs et al. (1983) failed to find significant differences among faster versus slower or more-experienced versus less-experienced runners in any biochemical parameter they measured; others have found differences. Fowler, Chowdhury, Pearson, Gardner, and Bratton (1962) and Schmidt and Schmidt (1969) stated that the elevation of enzyme activities depends on the duration and degree of exertion and that training lowers enzyme elevation after exercise. Noakes and Carter (1982) found that higher levels of training or previous ultramarathon racing experience was associated with less-elevated postexercise levels of enzyme than in novice runners.

Hansen et al. (1982) found that serum myoglobin values were higher in less-trained runners and decreased with more training. They concluded that superior training leads to less muscle cell membrane permeability during running, and consequently, less leakage of protein from muscle cells to the intravascular space.

General Discussion and Conclusions

There are many stresses involved in marathon running. Prolonged pounding of the feet on hard surfaces may cause trauma to local tissues.

Intense and protracted demand for substrate and oxygen delivery to working muscle presents a severe cardiorespiratory challenge, particularly for the poorly prepared, and for all runners under adverse environmental conditions. In addition, there is the emotional excitement of competition and often dehydration and hyperthermia. In response to exertion there are fluid shifts from the muscular to the intravascular, from the intravascular to the muscular, and from the lymphatic to the intravascular compartments. It is most remarkable that the homeostatic mechanisms of the trained runner function as well as they do to prevent more excessive deviations from the normal state despite the severe stresses of marathon running.

Exactly what all these changes in blood chemistry mean awaits further study. One thing, I believe, is clear—that marathon running induces *abnormal* blood chemistry values that are *normal* physiological responses to the stresses imposed. If one interpreted many of the results presented here as signs of disease, many of these athletes would be diagnosed as having anemia, liver disease, renal failure, myocardial ischemia, and even myocardial infarction.

The results presented here point out that the physician must thoroughly know the patient before drawing conclusions from a blood chemistry profile. An endurance athlete presenting for a routine medical examination after a long training run or a marathon race will have blood chemistry values that are different from nonrunners. CPK, LDH, ASAT, and ALAT values may remain elevated for weeks following a race. Without an adequate patient history—without knowledge of the patient's active life-style and training routine—the physician will simply not know how to interpret such disparate blood chemistry results.

In the event that a collapsed runner is taken to the emergency room, it behooves the well-prepared physician to know what to expect by way of blood chemistry tests after a marathon. "Normal" responses may then clearly stand out from "abnormal" responses, and much time may be saved in determining a course of treatment.

Some studies have observed differences between faster and slower runners, experienced and inexperienced, younger and older runners, and those running more compared with those running less weekly mileage. Others have not. We did not find many differences between male and female runners. It appears that physiological responses to long-distance running are relatively similar for all—the average participant as well as the elite performer.

References

Block, P., Van Rijmenant, M., Badjov, R., Van Melsem, A.Y., & Vogeleer, R. (1969). The effects of exhaustive effort on serum enzymes in man. In J.R. Poortmans (Ed.), *Biochemistry of Exercise* **Vol. 3** (pp. 259-267). Baltimore, MD: University Park Press.

Castenfors, J. (1977). Renal function during prolonged exercise. *Annals of the New York Academy of Sciences, 301*, 151-159.

Costill, D.L., & Fink, W.J. (1974). Plasma volume changes following exercise and thermal dehydration. *Journal of Applied Physiology, 37*, 521-525.

Dale, E., Gerlach, D.H., Martin, D.E. & Alexander, C.R. (1979). Physical fitness profiles and reproductive physiology of the female distance runner. *The Physician and Sportsmedicine, 7*(1), 83-95.

Dancaster, C.P. & Whereat, S.J. (1971). Fluid and electrolyte balance during the Comrades Marathon. *South African Medical Journal, 45*, 147-150.

Dickson, D.N., Dickinson, R.L., & Noakes, T.D. (1982). Effects of ultra-marathon training and racing on hematologic parameters and serum ferritin levels in well-trained athletes. *International Journal of Sports Medicine, 3*, 111-117.

Dill, D.B., & Costill, D.L. (1974). Calculation of percentage changes in volumes of blood, plasma, and red cells in dehydration. *Journal of Applied Physiology, 37*, 247-248.

Dressendorfer, R.H., Scaff, J.H., Jr., Wagner, J.O., & Gallup, J.D. (1977). Metabolic adjustments to marathon running in coronary patients. *Annals of the New York Academy of Sciences, 301*, 466-483.

Fowler, W.M., Jr., Chowdhury, S.R., Pearson, C.M., Gardner, G., & Bratton, R. (1962). Changes in serum levels after exercise in trained and untrained subjects. *Journal of Applied Physiology, 17*, 943-946.

Gilligan, D.R., Altschule, M.D., & Katersky, E.M. (1943). Physiological intravascular hemolysis of exercise. Hemoglobinemia and hemoglobinuria following cross-country runs. *Journal of Clinical Investigation, 22*, 859-869.

Hansen, K. Norregaard, Bjerre-Knudsen, J., Brodthagen, U., Jordal, R., & Paulev, P.-E. (1982). Muscle cell leakage due to long distance training. *European Journal of Applied Physiology, 48*, 177-188.

Hunter, J.B., & Critz, J.B. (1971). Effect of training on plasma enzyme levels in men. *Journal of Applied Physiology, 31*, 20-23.

Kolka, M.A., Stephenson, L.A., Witten, M., Fee, N., & Wilkerson, J.E., (1978). Blood, red cell, and plasma volume changes during long term recovery from marathon racing. *Medicine and Science in Sports, 10*, 61, (Abstract).

Krebs, P.S., Scully, B.C., & Zinkgraf, S.A. (1983). The acute and prolonged effects of marathon running on 20 blood parameters. *The Physician and Sportsmedicine, 11*(4), 66-73.

Magazanik, A., Shapiro, Y., Meytes, D., & Meytes, J. (1974). Enzyme blood levels and water balance during a marathon race. *Journal of Applied Physiology, 36*, 214-217.

Maron, M.B., Horvath, S.M., & Wilkerson, J.E. (1975). Acute blood biochemical alterations in response to marathon running. *European Journal of Applied Physiology, 34*, 173-181.

Maron, M.B., Horvath, S.M., & Wilkerson, J.E. (1977). Blood biochemical alterations during recovery from competitive marathon running. *European Journal of Applied Physiology, 36*, 231-238.

Martin, R.P., Haskell, W.L., & Wood, P.D. (1977). Blood chemistry and lipid profiles of elite distance runners. *Annals of the New York Academy of Sciences, 301*, 346-360.

McKechnie, J.K., Leary, W.P., & Joubert, S.M. (1967). Some electrocardiographic and biochemical changes in marathon runners. *South African Medical Journal, 41*, 722-725.

Myhre, L.G., Hartung, G.H., & Tucker, D.M. (1982). Plasma volume and blood metabolites in middle-aged runners during a warm-weather marathon. *European Journal of Applied Physiology, 48*, 227-240.

Noakes, T.D., & Carter, J.W. (1982). The responses of plasma biochemical parameters to a 56-km race in novice and experienced ultra-marathon runners. *European Journal of Applied Physiology, 49*, 179-186.

Riley, W.J., Pyke, F.S., Roberts, A.D., & England, J.F. (1975). The effect of long-distance running on some biochemical variables. *Clinica Chimica Acta, 65*, 83-89.

Robbins, S.L., & Angell, M. (1976). *Basic pathology.* Philadelphia, W.B. Saunders.

Rose, L.I., Bousser, J.E., & Cooper, K.H. (1970). Serum enzymes after marathon running. *Journal of Applied Physiology, 29*, 355-357.

Rose, L.I., Carroll, D.R., Lowe, S.L., Peterson, E.W., & Cooper, K.H. (1970). Serum electrolyte changes after marathon running. *Journal of Applied Physiology, 29*, 449-451.

Rose, L.I., Lowe, S.L., Carroll, D.R., Wolfson, S., & Cooper, K.H. (1970). Serum lactate dehydrogenase isoenzyme changes after muscular exertion. *Journal of Applied Physiology, 28*, 279-281.

Scheele, J., Herzog, W., Ritthaler, G., Wirth, A., & Weicker, H. (1979). Metabolic adaptation to prolonged exercise. *European Journal of Applied Physiology, 41*, 101-108.

Schmidt, E., & Schmidt, F.W. (1969). Enzyme modifications during activity. In J.R. Poortmans (Ed.), *Biochemistry of Exercise* Vol 3 (pp. 216-238). Baltimore, MD, University Park Press.

Senay, L.C., Jr. (1979). Effects of exercise in the heat on body fluid distribution. *Medicine and Science in Sports, 11*, 42-48.

Shapiro, Y., Magazanik, A., Sohar, E., & Reich, C.B. (1973). Serum enzyme changes in untrained subjects following a prolonged march. *Canadian Journal of Physiology and Pharmacology, 51*, 271-276.

Superko, H.R., Catlin, M.J., & Smith, J.L. (1979). Serum enzyme changes in prolonged endurance competition. *Medicine and Science in Sports, 11*, 89 (Abstract).

Thompson, P.D., Cullinane, E., Henderson, L.O., & Herbert, P.N. (1980). Acute effects of prolonged exercise on serum lipids. *Metabolism, 29*, 662-665.

Viru, A., & Korge, P. (1971). Metabolic processes and adrenocortical activity during marathon races. *Internationale Zeitschriff angewandte Physiologie,* **29**, 173-183.

Wells, C.L., Hecht, L.H., & Krahenbuhl, G.S. (1981). Physical characteristics and oxygen utilization of male and female marathon runners. *Research Quarterly for Exercise and Sport,* **52**, 281-285.

Wells, C.L., Stern, J.R., & Hecht, L.H. (1982). Hematological changes following a marathon race in male and female runners. *European Journal of Applied Physiology,* **48**, 41-49.

Williams, M.H., & Ward, A.J. (1977). Hematological changes elicited by prolonged intermittent aerobic exercise. *Research Quarterly,* **48**, 606-616.

Wilkerson, J.E., Gutin, B., & Horvath, S.M. (1977). Exercise-induced changes in blood, red cell, and plasma volumes in man. *Medicine and Science in Sports,* **9**, 155-158.

Wilkerson, J.E., Kolka, M.A., & Stephenson, L.A. (1979). Exercise-induced leukocytosis during a competitive marathon. *Medicine and Science in Sports,* **11**, 99 (Abstract).

Winer, B.J. (1971). *Statistical principles in experimental design.* New York: McGraw Hill.

7 Gender Differences in Heat Tolerance: Fact or Fiction?

Barbara L. Drinkwater
Pacific Medical Center

One of the major challenges facing endurance athletes, whether in training or competition, is the dissipation of the heat produced during intense physical activity. When the environment compounds the problem, either by adding to the thermal load or by restricting heat loss, the situation can become a serious threat to the welfare of the athlete. For many years it was presumed that women were less able to tolerate this combination of stressors (Burse, 1979). This assumption was based on the results of laboratory studies of sex differences in thermoregulation, which reported that women had higher core temperatures, higher heart rates, lower sweat production, and lower tolerance times than men when both performed the same task in hot environments.

Now that it is recognized that relative work load, not absolute work load, determines many of the indices of heat strain, it is evident that differences in cardiovascular fitness rather than gender could have accounted for the apparent sex differences. The same factor may play a role in the apparent decline in heat tolerance with aging. The success of women such as Sister Marion Irvine, who qualified for the first Olympic Marathon Trials for women at age 54, suggests a need to reevaluate the relationship between age and thermoregulation.

If indeed there are differences in heat tolerance between men and women or younger and older adults, one would expect to find these differences reflected in the components of the thermal balance equation:

$$S = M \pm (R + C + K) - E \pm W.$$

How might an individual's gender or age affect heat storage (S) by altering the balance between metabolic heat production (M), heat transfer by radiation (R), convection (C), and conduction (K), evaporative heat loss (E), and heat expended in or gained by positive or negative work (W)?

Two possibilities exist:

(1) Although there is differential utilization of avenues for heat loss or heat gain may be used, the end result, S, is the same, or

(2) There are quantitive differences in the amount of heat produced or exchanged, which result in different values for S.

For example, it has been suggested that women rely more on convective heat loss when $\overline{T}_{sk} > T_a$ because of their higher surface area to mass ratio (A_D/w), while men depend more on evaporative heat loss (Shapiro, Pandolf, Avellini, Pimental, & Goldman, 1981). Under favorable environmental conditions, S could be the same for both sexes. However, when young males show less heat strain than either women or older men under the same stress, the implication is that they are losing more heat by (R + C) and/or E and storing less. When the greatest discrepancy between groups was found in sweat rate, hypotheses were advanced that neural degeneration might account for the aging effect (Wagner, Robinson, Tzankoff, & Marino, 1972), while hormonal differences could be a major factor in the lower sweat rate of females (Kawahata, 1960; Haslag & Hertzman, 1965). However, if one looks behind the symbols of the thermal balance equation to the physiological responses they represent, it is obvious that factors other than gender and age can account for the large inter-individual variability in heat tolerance observed in any population. The purpose of this review is to evaluate recent research on one such factor, maximal aerobic power ($\dot{V}O_2max$), when comparing the thermoregulatory response of individuals who differ in sex and in age.

Sex Differences in Thermoregulation

The observation by a number of investigators (Kawahata, 1960; Wyndham, Morrison, & Williams, 1965; Morimoto, Slabochova, Naman, & Sargent, 1967) that women sweat less than men under comparable conditions of heat stress has been accepted by many as a basic sex difference in thermoregulation that explains why women had higher core temperatures (Tc), higher heart rates (HR), and lower tolerance times than men in those studies. Although Åstrand (1960) had already noted that core temperature was more closely related to relative work load (% $\dot{V}O_2max$) than to absolute exercise intensity, these early studies (Wyndham et al., 1965; Morimoto et al., 1967) assigned the same task to both men and women. Because it is a reasonable assumption that women were less active and less fit than men in the 1960s, it is probable that the response to heat stress was confounded by the response to exercise.

With the advantage of hindsight, it is also apparent that fitness levels ($\dot{V}O_2max$) affected the thermoregulatory response when men and women were resting in the heat (Fox, Löfstedt, Woodward, Eriksson, & Werkstrom, 1969). Both the sensitivity and capacity of the sweating response are enhanced by physical training. The fit individual not only begins sweating at a lower Tc but produces more sweat at any given level of internal temperature (Henane, Flandrois, & Charbonnier, 1977; Nadel, Pandolf, Roberts, & Stolwijk, 1974).

When Japanese female athletes (FA) and female (FNA) and male (MNA) nonathletes were observed in a 32° C environment with their legs submerged in a 42° C water bath, the threshold Tc for onset of sweating was 0.3° C less for FA than for either FNA or MNA (Kobayashi, Ando, Okuda, Takaba, & Ohara, 1980). The FA also had a higher sweat rate ($\dot{m}_{sw}$) than FNA or MNA at any given Tc and lower HRs and Tcs during the entire 2-hour period.

It is evident that habitual vigorous exercise modifies the thermoregulatory response to heat stress. Because this factor was not considered in the experimental design of the earlier (<1976) studies of sex differences in thermoregulation, it is probable that many of the apparent sex-related physiological differences were associated with differences in aerobic power rather than gender. It was not always the women who suffered in comparison with the men. In one study (Weinman, Slabochova, Bernauer, Morimoto, & Sargent, 1967) physically active women were compared with less-active men, and the males had the higher HR and Tc in spite of having higher sweat rates. This group (Weinman, et al.) was the first to suggest that the level of physical fitness might account for many of the apparent sex differences in response to heat stress.

In effect, physical training as well as heat acclimation shifts the setpoint for the initiation of thermoregulatory responses (Gisolfi & Weigner, 1984). Assigning exercise at the same relative intensity (% $\dot{V}O_2$max) to individuals who differ only slightly in fitness levels may compensate for this shift. However, when two groups have markedly different $\dot{V}O_2$max values, the active life-style of the individuals with a higher aerobic power results in physiological changes whose impact on heat tolerance is not nullified by assigning the same relative workload to each group. This became apparent when female athletes and nonathletes exercised at $\sim$30% $\dot{V}O_2$max in mild heat (28° C, 12.6 torr vp), humid heat (35° C, 28 torr vp), and dry heat (48° C, 8.7 torr vp) (Drinkwater, Denton, Kupprat, Talag, & Horvath, 1976). Although there were no significant differences between groups in HR or Tc during exercise in 28° C or 35° C, nonathletes were unable to maintain stroke volume (SV) and cardiac output ($\dot{Q}$) by the 45th min of exercise in 48° C. Within 10 min, average Tc for this group reached 39° C, the criteria level for removal from the chamber. The mean Tc for athletes reached this point only after 120 min in the chamber.

The benefits of endurance training for female athletes include a lower resting Tc and HR, a larger plasma volume, more influx of plasma protein into the vascular space and less decrease in plasma volume during exercise in the heat, and an earlier onset of sweating (Drinkwater, Kupprat, Denton, & Horvath, 1977). The improvement in cardiovascular stability, heat exchange, and tolerance time is similar to that reported for males following conditioning programs (Pandolf, 1979). The extent of improvement in exercise-heat tolerance as a result of physical training depends on the intensity and duration of training (Pandolf, 1979) and the type of activity (Henane et al., 1977). Swimmers, for example, tolerated heat stress better than sedentary males, but their sweat production was significantly lower than that of cross-country skiers (Henane et al.). The implication is that an elevated core temperature during training is required to increase the sweating response. The same requirement appears to hold for females. When women were assigned to either a heat acclimation or a training group, all demonstrated an improvement in heat tolerance after exercising at 50% $\dot{V}O_2$max for 9 days in either a hot (48° C) or cool (23° C) environment (Kupprat, Drinkwater, & Horvath, 1980). The improvement in Tc, HR, $\overline{T}_{sk}$, and evaporative heat loss of the training group averaged 45% of the change observed in the acclimation group, a figure close to the average 50% improvement in heat tolerance noted for men following a training program (Pandolf). The major difference between the two groups was in evaporative heat loss ($\dot{m}_{sw}$). The training group, whose exercise Tc was maintained at or below 38.5° C, increased $\dot{m}_{sw}$ by 2.3W/m²; the acclimation group; 28.0 W/m².

The implication from these studies is that an experimental design that does not include aerobic power and training regimens as factors cannot answer questions regarding sex differences in thermoregulation. In essence, this precludes citing most studies done before the mid or late 1970s as evidence that women are less able to tolerate exercise in the heat than men.

Initial efforts to correct this design deficiency relied on assigning the same relative exercise intensity to males and females without matching groups for $\dot{V}O_2$max. Paolone, Wells, and Kelly (1978) tested nonacclimated men and women at 50% $\dot{V}O_2$max in a neutral (25° C), warm (32° C), and hot (40° C) environment with humidity constant at 50% to 55%. Although the men had a greater evaporative weight loss and total sweat rate in all three environments, they also had higher exercise heart rates ($\overline{X} \Delta = 12.3$ bpm). There were no significant differences in Tc or $\overline{T}_{sk}$. Wells (1980) followed up with a similar study using acclimated subjects and exposing them to the natural environment stress of the Arizona desert (39.1° C). In this dry heat there were no differences between groups in either Tc, HR, ($\dot{m}_{sw}$), or evaporative weight loss. Women had a higher $\overline{T}_{sk}$ than the men during the 40-min exercise period. Although neither study matched subjects for $\dot{V}O_2$max, the difference between the men and women was $\curvearrowright$11% in ml O_2 • kg^{-1} • min^{-1} in both. However, the men in the Paolone et al. (1978) study were producing $\curvearrowright$25% more metabolic heat (W/m²) than the women, while in the Wells study (1980) the difference was only 12%. Because sweat rate is directly related to metabolic heat production, this difference may explain why Paolone et al. found a sex difference in evaporative weight loss and Wells did not. On the other hand, the state of acclimation of the Arizona subjects or the difference in relative humidity between the two locations might have affected the results.

In 1979, Davies looked at the ability of male and female athletes to dissipate metabolic heat when exercising at 76% $\dot{V}O_2$max for 60 min in a cool environment (21° C, 50% rh). There were no significant differences between the sexes in Tc or $\overline{T}_{sk}$. In this report, the higher $\dot{m}_{sw}$ of the male athletes was shown to be directly proportional to total heat production. When $\dot{m}_{sw}$ was expressed as a percent of maximal sweating capacity (%$\dot{m}_{sw}$ max), it was linearly related to Tc and did not differ between the sexes. Davies concluded that thermoregulatory function was not related to sex. An interesting aspect of this report was a comparison of the female athletes ($\dot{V}O_2$max = 58.7 ml • min^{-1})

with four active male nonathletes ($\dot{V}O_2$max $= 58.1$ ml $\cdot$ kg^{-1} $\cdot$ min^{-1}). Metabolic heat production for the men averaged 549 W/m^2; for the women, 529 W/m^2. In this cool dry environment, $\dot{m}_{sw}$ for the women (279 W/m^2) was approximately equal to that of the men (269 W/m^2). No differences were apparent in either Tc or $\overline{T}_{sk}$. On the basis of Davies' (1979) study it appears that active men and women matched in $\dot{V}O_2$max and exercising for 60 min in a cool environment respond almost identically in dissipating metabolic heat. Does this similarity persist with the imposition of an external heat load as well?

Avellini, Kamon, and Krajewski (1980) matched four men and four women for $\dot{V}O_2$max (ml $\cdot$ kg LBM^{-1} $\cdot$ min^{-1}) and for A_D/wt before exercising them at $\sim$30% $\dot{V}O_2$max in humid heat (36°/30° C, db/wb) for 3 hrs. Although the men had higher sweat rates, their Tc and HR were higher and tolerance times lower than those of the women. The authors (Avellini et al.) suggested that women might have a physiological advantage in humid heat because they were able to accomplish the same amount of work as men with less indication of strain and less loss of body fluids. A companion paper (Frye & Kamon, 1981) explored the possibility that this advantage would be lost in dry heat (48°/25° C, db/wb), where the capacity for evaporative heat loss would be much higher and men's higher $\dot{m}_{sw}$ might be advantageous. Although the sexes were matched on $\dot{V}O_2$max (ml $\cdot$ kg $^{-1}$ $\cdot$ min^{-1}) A_D, and A_D/wt, and worked at the same relative intensity ($\sim$30% $\dot{V}O_2$max), the men had longer tolerance times (121 vs 82 min) and a higher $\dot{m}_{sw}$. The rate of increase in Tc was significantly higher for women, so that by 70 min of exercise their Tc had reached 38.8° C while the men's was only 38.1° C. Although final HR and $\overline{T}_{sk}$ were the same for both groups, the men exercised longer before reaching those values. The results appeared to support the authors' hypothesis that men would have lower indices of heat strain than women when ambient conditions permitted free evaporation of sweat.

However, Horstman and Christensen (1982) were unable to fully corroborate these results when exercising men and women at 40% $\dot{V}O_2$max in a similar environment (45°/23° C, db/wb). Although women's HRs averaged $\sim$15 bpm higher than the men's, there were no significant differences in the rate of increase for Tc, HR, or $\dot{m}_{sw}$/ΔTc. Performance times were slightly less for men (74 min) than for women (83 min), although the men took advantage of the evaporative potential of the environment by producing more sweat (596 g $\cdot$ m^{-2} $\cdot$ hr^{-1}) than the women (461 g $\cdot$ m^{-2} $\cdot$ hr^{-1}).

In all three of the foregoing studies (Avellini et al., 1980; Frye & Kamon, 1981; Horstman & Christensen, 1982) the acute exposure to exercise in the respective environments was followed by a period of acclimation. In humid heat (Avellini, et al.), the men increased $\dot{m}_{sw}$ significantly more than women but completed the 3 hrs of exercise with a higher Tc (Δ 0.3° C) and HR (Δ 10 bpm). Their marked increase in $\dot{m}_{sw}$ in an environment where maximal evaporation (Emax) was limited by high humidity was not effective in improving dissipation of heat. In the Frye and Kamon study (1981) the apparent advantage of the higher male $\dot{m}_{sw}$ in the dry heat disappeared after 8-9 days of acclimation.

During postacclimation heat stress tests, men and women had the same $\dot{m}_{sw}$, $\Delta\dot{m}_{sw}/\Delta Tc$, and sweating threshold. Indices of heat strain, Tc, HR, $\overline{T}_{sk}$, and tolerance time were the same for both sexes. Women were able to achieve parity with the men by increasing their $\dot{m}_{sw}$ by 41% during acclimation, while the men added only 10% to their sweat production.

The dry heat was not an advantage for acclimated men in the Horstman and Christensen (1982) study. In spite of maintaining a higher $\dot{m}_{sw}$, the men had lower tolerance times (100 vs 120 min), a lower $\dot{m}_{sw}/\Delta Tc$, and a larger increase in Tc. Neither final HR nor ΔHR differed between the sexes. Under similar conditions to those used in the Frye and Kamon study, the women had much less increase in $\dot{m}_{sw}$ ($\sim$ 12%), while the men had slightly more ($\sim$ 16%). On the basis of these two studies (Frye & Kamon, 1981; Horstman & Christensen, 1982) one would conclude that any advantage a high $\dot{m}_{sw}$ confers on males in dry heat disappears after acclimation.

The importance of considering aerobic power, activity patterns, and A_D/wt in the experimental design of heat stress studies is illustrated in a series of reports coming out of the Natick laboratories between 1980 and 1982. The physiological responses of nine women ($\dot{V}O_2max = 40.5$ ml $\cdot$ kg^{-1} $\cdot$ min^{-1}) and 10 men ($\dot{V}O_2max = 52.3$ ml $\cdot$ kg^{-1} $\cdot$ min^{-1}) were recorded during 2-hr acclimation periods in a 49° C, 20% rh environment for 6 days (Shapiro, Pandolf, & Goldman, 1980), during a 4-hr exercise period in the same environment following acclimation (Avellini, Shapiro, Pandolf, Pimental, & Goldman, 1980), and in five additional thermal environments after acclimation in 49° C, 20% rh (Shapiro, Pandolf, Avellini, Pimental, & Goldman, 1980). Data from the latter study were then used to examine thermal balance and heat exchange when expressed relative to body weight or body surface area. (Shapiro, Pandolf, Avellini, Pimental, & Goldman, 1981).

In the original acclimation study (Shapiro, Pandolf, & Goldman, 1980) the authors concluded that women have a higher thermoregulatory setpoint than men because their $\overline{T}_{sk}$ and Tc were higher both before and after acclimation. The difference in fitness levels, as reflected by the 11.8 ml $\cdot$ kg^{-1} $\cdot$ min^{-1} difference in $\dot{V}O_2max$, was not considered a major factor in these results. When exposure time was extended to 4 hrs for these same subjects, there were no significant differences in Tc at any point in the 4-hr period (Avellini et al., 1980). The higher HR of the women throughout the third and fourth hour was attributed to the higher relative workload of the women (36% $\dot{V}O_2max$) compared with the men's exercise intensity (29% $\dot{V}O_2max$). As in the acclimation period, $\overline{T}_{sk}$ was higher for women than men, while E $_{sw}$ was less. When the subjects were divided into "most fit" and "least fit" categories, the least fit males were exercising at 31.3% $\dot{V}O_2max$. When compared with the most fit females walking at 32.9% $\dot{V}O_2max$, the men's Tc (38.2° C) and HR (144 bpm) were the same as those of the women (38.2° C and 145 bpm). This observation suggests that the statement in the earlier paper (Shapiro, Pandolf, & Goldman) that fitness levels did not markedly influence the results may have been in error.

When these men and women repeated the 2-hr protocol in several hot-dry (HD) and hot-wet (HW) environments, the women had a higher Tc and HR in the most severe HD conditions and a lower Tc in the most severe HW environment (Shapiro, Pandolf, Avellini, Pimental, & Goldman, 1980). The authors suggest that the higher A_D/wt of the women was a disadvantage in HD climates because it facilitated heat gain via R + C and an advantage in HW conditions when R + C is the most important avenue for heat dissipation. Yet when the same authors (Shapiro et al., 1981) expressed heat exchange components relative to body surface area (m²), they concluded that the larger A_D/wt of the females was not a disadvantage in HD conditions because their higher $\overline{T}_{sk}$ reduced heat gain from the environment via R + C by minimizing the $(\overline{T}_{sk} - Ta)$ gradient.

Part of the contradictions regarding sex differences in thermoregulation in the literature can be explained by the failure of some investigators to consider the effect of physical training on thermoregulatory function. The most obvious error is the failure to assign the same relative workload to all subjects. More subtle is the effect of matching women and men for $\dot{V}O_2$max, correcting for body weight (ml · kg⁻¹ · min⁻¹) or weight plus fat (ml · kg LBM⁻¹) without regard to other factors that may account for sex differences in maximal aerobic power. Were the men ($\dot{V}O_2$max = 64.2 m. · kg LBM⁻¹) and women ($\dot{V}O_2$max = 65.7 ml · kg LBM⁻¹) in the Avellini, Damon, and Krajewski (1980) study actually matched on fitness? Cureton (1981) suggests that a difference of ∿ 5% in $\dot{V}O_2$max (ml · kg LBM⁻¹ · min⁻¹) is necessary to account for inherent biological differences between the sexes, such as hemoglobin levels, which affect $\dot{V}O_2$max. If so, one reason for the higher Tc, higher HR, and lower tolerance time of the men in the Avellini et al. study might be that the women were actually at a higher level of training. More thought must be given to the problem of equating men and women on fitness levels in studies where differences in physical conditioning can be a confounding factor in the results.

Another potential problem is the small sample size in some studies. Frye & Kamon (1981) found no significant difference in the final HRs of men (106.2 bpm) and women (120.6 bpm) exercising 3 hrs in dry heat. A similar difference between men (117.0 bpm) and women (130.1 bpm) in the Shapiro, Pandolf, Avellini, Pimental, and Goldman (1980) study was significant. The contradiction in results is an example of how sample size affects statistical results. The Shapiro et al. study included nine females and 10 males; the Frye and Kamon study, four of each. Although the absolute difference in HR was almost identical, the difference was significant only in the study with the larger sample size.

On the basis of current information regarding the thermoregulatory responses of men and women exercising in hot-humid or hot-dry environments, female athletes should be at no greater risk than male athletes when competing in the heat. Before acclimation women may actually have an advantage in hot-humid conditions because their larger A_D/wt enhances heat loss via R + C when evaporative heat loss is limited. Results from studies of sex differences in hot-dry environments are mixed, and further study is warranted. However, following acclimation both men and women increased tolerance times, $\dot{m}_{sw}$, $\dot{m}_{sw}/\Delta Tre$, and decreased HR and $\overline{T}_{sk}$. When sex differences in response were apparent, they favored the women when both groups were exercising at the same $\%\dot{V}O_2max$. Fitness level and state of heat acclimation are more important than gender in assessing the adequacy of any guidelines designed to protect athletes from heat injury.

Age Differences in Thermoregulation

The thermoregulatory response of many older adults to exercise in hot environments has been described as inadequate to meet the demands of the thermal load imposed by metabolic heat production and environmental heat stress (Drinkwater & Horvath, 1979; Löfstedt, 1966; Wagner, Robinson, Tzankoff, & Marino, 1972). As morbidity and mortality rates during periodic heat waves can attest, older individuals are more at risk in the heat even without the added stress of physical activity (U.S. Dept. of Health and Human Services, 1981). Two explanations have been suggested to explain the apparent effect of aging on heat tolerance. Some investigators (Hellon & Lind, 1956; Hellon, Lind, & Weiner, 1956; Löfstedt, 1966; Wagner et al., 1972) believe an age-related decrease in the sensitivity and capacity of the sweating mechanism is responsible. Others (Dill & Consolazio, 1962; Dill, Kasch, Yousef, Saholt, & Wolfenbarger, 1975; Drinkwater & Horvath, 1979) have suggested that an inadequate cardiovascular response related to a decrease in physical fitness is the cause. In a review of thermoregulation and aging, Drinkwater and Horvath (1979) pointed out some of the difficulties involved in matching younger and older adults for aerobic power, because the same $\dot{V}O_2max$ can represent quite different levels of habitual activity for a 20-year-old and a 70-year-old individual. There are, however, some design and statistical techniques that can assist the investigator in determining what thermoregulatory responses are related to age and which can be explained by differences in physical fitness.

When 38 nonacclimated females aged 12 to 68 years exercised in three hot environments at $\sim 30\% \dot{V}O_2max$, a multiple regression technique was used to determine what factors were related to heat tolerance (Drinkwater & Horvath, 1979). Age did not prove to be a significant predictor. The important factors were the cardiac response to heat-exercise stress, the adequacy of the sweating response, and the ability to shift plasma into the cardiovascular space. Since all three factors are known to be related to physical fitness, the authors (Drinkwater & Horvath) suggested that the decrement in $\dot{V}O_2max$ with age could be an important factor in explaining the apparent decrease in heat tolerance of the older age-group. During the same year, Davies (1979) compared the thermoregulatory function of young male athletes (31.8 years) and older male athletes (60.2 years) exercising at 76% $\dot{V}O_2$max in a mild environment (21°/15° C, db/wb). Core temperature and $\overline{T}_{sk}$ were the same for both groups. Because the younger men were exercising at a higher absolute metabolic rate, their $\dot{m}_{sw}$ was also greater W/m². However, when $\dot{m}_{sw}$ was plotted relative to $\dot{m}_{sw}$ max, there were no significant differences between age-groups. Davies concluded that the differences in temperature regulation ascribed to age in previous studies could be explained by differences in exercise capacity and suggested that regular physical activity might even diminish the risks older individuals face for hyperthermia.

Gonzales, Berglund, and Stolwijk (1980) also concluded that thermo-regulatory responses are more closely related to physical fitness than to age. They exposed males and females aged 8 to 67 years to thermal transients between 9° C and 50° C and found that an index of ability to compensate for heat stress effectively ($\Delta E_{sk}/\Delta Tc$) was more closely related to $\dot{V}O_2$max than age.

Because several studies (Hellon & Lind, 1956; Hellon, Lind, & Weiner, 1956; Löfstedt, 1966; Wagner et al., 1972) had suggested that older individuals not only sweat less but have a delayed onset of sweating, Drinkwater, Bedi, Loucks, Roche and Horvath (1982) examined the sweating sensitivity and capacity of younger and older women at rest in a hot-dry environment (40° C, 22.2 torr vp). Although there was a significant difference in $\dot{V}O_2$max between the older (31.5 ml • kg^{-1} • min^{-1}) and younger (46.8 ml • kg^{-1} • min^{-1}) groups, nine of the ten older women were physically active on a regular basis. There were no differences between age-groups in time for onset of sweating or the Tc threshold for sweating. Regional $\dot{m}_{sw}$ at five sites, E_{sw}, HR, Tc, forearm blood flow, and plasma volume shifts were the same for both age-groups. None of the thermoregulatory responses were related to age, but $\dot{m}_{sw}$ was significantly related to $\dot{V}O_2$max.

The same investigators (unpublished observations) examined the thermo-regulatory responses of similar age-groups performing light (60 W) work on a cycle ergometer in the same thermal environment. Because the emphasis of the investigation was on the sweating response, all women exercised at the same absolute work load. It was expected that those with lower levels of $\dot{V}O_2$max would have higher HRs and Tcs and lower tolerance times, and indeed they did. However, time and Tc at onset of sweating as well as E_{sw} were the same for younger and older women. It was concluded that some factor related to $\dot{V}O_2$max, not aging, is associated with the decrease in heat tolerance observed in some older individuals.

When two discrete groups such as male and female or young and old differ in their response to some external stressor, the tendency is to ascribe that difference to the most obvious characteristic identifying those groups—in this case sex and age. As recent studies have shown, the obvious conclusion is not always the scientifically sound conclusion. The less-obvious factors may play a more important role in dictating the physiological response. In the area of thermal regulation, that factor is physical conditioning. Neither female nor masters athletes should be more at risk than young male athletes when competing in hot environments.

References

Åstrand, I. (1960). Aerobic work capacity in men and women with special reference to age. *Acta Physiologica Scandinavica*, **49**, Supplement 169.

Avellini, B.A., Kamon, E., & Krajewski, J.T. (1980). Physiological responses of physically fit men and women to acclimation to humid heat. *Journal of Applied Physiology: Respiratory, Environmental, and Exercise Physiology*, **49**, 254-261.

Avellini, B.A., Shapiro, Y., Pandolf, K.B., Pimental, N.A., & Goldman, R.F. (1980). Physiological responses of men and women to prolonged dry heat exposure. *Aviation, Space, and Environmental Medicine*, **51**, 1081-1085.

Burse, R.L. (1979). Sex differences in thermoregulatory response to heat and cold stress. *Human Factors*, **21**, 687-699.

Buskirk, E. (1977). Temperature regulation with exercise. *Exercise and Sport Sciences Reviews*, **5**, 45-88.

Cureton, K.J. (1981). Matching of male and female subjects using $\dot{V}O_2$max. *Research Quarterly for Exercise and Sport*, **52**, 264-268.

Davies, C.T.M. (1979). Thermoregulation during exercise in relation to sex and age. *European Journal of Applied Physiology*, **42**, 71-79.

Dill, D.B., & Consolazio, C.F. (1962). Responses to exercise as related to age and experimental temperature. *Journal of Applied Physiology*, **17**, 645-648.

Dill, D.B., Kasch, F.W., Yousef, M.K., Soholt, L.F., & Wolfenbarger, D.L. (1975). Cardiovascular responses and temperature regulation in relation to age. *Australian Journal of Sports Medicine*, **7**, 99-106.

Drinkwater, B.L., Bedi, J.F., Loucks, A.B., Roche, S., & Horvath, S.M. (1982). Sweating sensitivity and capacity of women in relation to age. *Journal of Applied Physiology: Respiratory, Environmental, and Exercise Physiology*, **53**, 671-676.

Drinkwater, B.L., Denton, J.E., Kupprat, I.C., Talag, T.S., & Horvath, S.M. (1976). Aerobic power as a factor in women's response to work in hot environments. *Journal of Applied Physiology*, **41**, 815-821.

Drinkwater, B.L., & Horvath, S.M. (1979). Heat tolerance and aging. *Medicine and Science in Sports*, **11**, 49-55.

Drinkwater, B.L., Kupprat, I.C., Denton, J.E., & Horvath, S.M. (1977). Heat tolerance of female distance runners. *Annals of the New York Academy of Science*, **301**, 777-792.

Fox, R.H., Löfstedt, B.E., Woodward, P.M., Eriksson, E., & Werkstrom, B. (1969). Comparison of thermoregulatory function in men and women. *Journal of Applied Physiology,* **26**, 444-453.

Frye, A.J., & Kamon, E. (1981). Responses to dry heat of men and women with similar aerobic capacities. *Journal of Applied Physiology: Respiratory, Environmental, and Exercise Physiology,* **50**, 65-70.

Gisolfi, C.V., & Wenger, C.B. (1984). Temperature regulation during exercise: Old concepts, new ideas. In R.J. Terjung, (Ed.), *Exercise and Sport Sciences Reviews* (pp. 339-372). Lexington, MA: The Collamore Press.

Gonzales, R.R., Berglund, L.G., & Stolwijk, J.A.J. (1980). Thermoregulation in humans of different ages during thermal transients. In Z. Szelenyi & M. Szekely (Eds.), *Satellite of 28th International Congress of Physiological Sciences, 1980* (pp. 357-361). Copenhagen: August Krogh Institute, University of Copenhagen.

Haslag, W.M. & Hertzman, A.B. (1965). Temperature regulation in young women. *Journal of Applied Physiology,* **20**, 1283-1288.

Hellon, R.F., & Lind, A.R. (1956). Observations on the activity of sweat glands with special reference to the influence of aging. *Journal of Physiology,* **133**, 132-144.

Hellon, R.F., Lind, A.R., & Weiner, J.S. (1956). The physiological reactions of men of two age groups to a hot environment. *Journal of Physiology,* **133**, 118-131.

Henane, R., Flandrois, R., & Charbonnier, J.P. (1977). Increase in sweating sensitivity by endurance conditioning in man. *Journal of Applied Physiology: Respiratory, Environmental, and Exercise Physiology,* **43**, 822-828.

Horstman, D.H., & Christensen, E. (1982). Acclimatization to dry heat: Active men vs active women. *Journal of Applied Physiology: Respiratory, Environmental, and Exercise Physiology,* **52**, 825-831.

Kawahata, A. (1960). Sex differences in sweating. In H. Yoshimura, K. Ogata, & S. Itoh (Eds.), *Essential problems in climatic physiology* (pp. 169-195). Kyoto: Nankodo.

Kobayashi, Y., Ando, Y., Okuda, N., Takaba, S., & Ohara, K. (1980). Effects of endurance training in thermoregulation in females. *Medicine and Science in Sports,* **12**, 361-364.

Kupprat, I.C., Drinkwater, B.L., & Horvath, S.M. (1980). Interaction of exercise and ambient environment during heat acclimation. *Hungarian Review of Sports Medicine,* **21**, 5-16.

Löfstedt, B. (1966). *Human heat tolerance.* Lund, Sweden: Department of Hygiene, University of Lund.

Morimoto, T., Slabochova, Z., Naman, R.K., & Sargent II, F. (1967). Sex differences in physiological reactions to thermal stress. *Journal of Applied Physiology,* **22**, 526-532.

Nadel, E.R., Pandolf, K.B., Roberts, M.F., & Stolwijk, J.A.J. (1974). Mechanics of thermal acclimation to exercise and heat. *Journal of Applied Physiology, 37*, 515-520.

Pandolf, K.B., (1979). Effects of physical training and cardiorespiratory physical fitness on exercise-heat tolerance: Recent observations. *Medicine and Science in Sports, 11*, 60-65.

Paolone, A.M., Wells, C.L., & Kelly, G.T. (1978). Sexual variations in thermoregulation during heat stress. *Aviation, Space, and Environmental Medicine, 49*, 715-719.

Shapiro, Y., Pandolf, K.B., Avellini, B.A., Pimental, N.A., & Goldman, R.F. (1980). Physiological responses of men and women to humid and dry heat. *Journal of Applied Physiology: Respiratory, Environmental, and Exercise Physiology, 49*, 1-8.

Shapiro, Y., Pandolf, K.B., Avellini, B.A., Pimental, N.A., & Goldman, R.F. (1981). Heat balance and transfer in men and women exercising in hot-dry and hot-wet conditions. *Ergonomics, 24*, 375-386.

Shapiro, Y., Pandolf, K.B., & Goldman, R.F. (1980). Sex differences in acclimation in a hot-dry environment. *Ergonomics, 23*, 635-642.

U.S. Department of Health and Human Services. (1981). Heatstroke. In United States, 1980, *Morbidity and Mortality Weekly Reports, 30*, 272-279. Washington, D.C.: U.S. Government Printing Office.

Wagner, J.A., Robinson, S., Tzankoff, S.P., & Marino, R.P. (1972). Heat tolerance and acclimatization to work in the heat in relation to age. *Journal of Applied Physiology, 33*, 616-622.

Weinman, K.P., Slabochova, Z., Bernauer, E.M., Morimoto, T., and Sargent II, F. (1967). Reactions of men and women to repeated exposure to humid heat. *Journal of Applied Physiology, 22*, 533-538.

Wells, C.L. (1980). Responses of physically active and acclimatized men and women to exercise in a desert environment. *Medicine and Science in Sports and Exercise, 12*, 9-13.

Wyndham, C.H., Morrison, J.F., & Williams, C.G. (1965). Heat reactions of male and female Caucasians. *Journal of Applied Physiology, 20*, 357-364.

8 Athletic Amenorrhea

Charlotte Feicht Sanborn
University of Denver

Wiltz W. Wagner, Jr.
Indiana University School of Medicine

In the past 20 years the number of women participating in endurance sports has increased dramatically. Female athletes are competing not only in marathons but in triathlons and ultramarathons. The latter events can be more than 100 miles of continuous, grueling physical work. Concern for the gynecological consequences of such strenuous activity has increased as reports of menstrual irregularities among female athletes have continued to rise. In fact, the cessation of menses, amenorrhea, has been found in athletes. To understand athletic amenorrhea, it is important to elucidate the following five aspects: its prevalence, its etiology, its reversibility, whether it is adaptive, and whether it has any harmful effects.

Prevalence of Athletic Amenorrhea

More than 2 decades ago, studies (Bausenwein, 1954; Erdelyi, 1963) introduced data indicating that training might be associated with menstrual irregularities. In 1954, Bausenwein compared 47 Olympic athletes to 70 physical education students. Irregular menstrual cycles were reported to be high among the Olympic athletes (12.8 %). Anecdotes were also provided of athletes whose menstrual irregularities were believed to coincide with training and competition.

Erdelyi (1963) was the first to report a possible association between intense training and amenorrhea. In a survey of 557 Hungarian female athletes, "unfavorable" menstrual cycle changes occurred in 62 (11%) of the sample. Some of the menstrual disorders listed were dysmenorrhea, irregular periods, and amenorrhea. Amenorrhea occurred more frequently in athletes who participated in strenuous activities such as tennis, rowing, and skiing. An association was also noticed between age and menstrual irregularities. A higher prevalence was found in the young athletes between 15 and 17 years of age than in those 18 and older.

Table 1   Prevalence of Secondary Amenorrhea

POPULATION	N	PERCENT	DEFINITION	REFERENCE
Controls				
College	500	2.3	>2 months no periods	Drew, 1961
Swedes	2000	3.3	<3 periods per year	Fries, Nillius and Peterson, 1974
Runners				
x-country	128	24.0	≤3 periods per year	Feicht, et al., 1978
x-country	38	44.7	no periods previous 3 months	Wakat, Sweeney and Rogol, 1982
>30 mpw	89	34.0	no definition provided	Dale, Gerlach, and Wilhite, 1979
5 to 30 mpw	22	23.0	no definition provided	Dale, Gerlach, and Wilhite, 1979
N.Y. Marathon	270	1.0	<1 period previous 10 months	Shangold and Levine, 1982
Joggers	885	6.0	no definition provided	Speroff and Redwine, 1980
Marathon	237	25.7	≤3 periods per year	Sanborn, Martin and Wagner, 1982
Ballet Dancers				
Students	69	18.8	at least 3 months no periods	Frisch, Wychak, and Vincent, 1980
Professional (29) + Students (5)	34	44.0	at least 3 months no periods	Calabrese, et al., 1983
Professional	32	36.7	at least 3 months no periods	Cohen, et al., 1982
Athletes				
College Varsity	140	12.1	no periods previous 3 months or < 4 periods per year	Carlberg, et al., 1983
Swimmers	197	12.3	≤3 periods per year	Sanborn, Martin and Wagner, 1982
Cyclists	33	12.1	≤3 periods per year	Sanborn, Martin and Wagner, 1982

Only recently, however, has amenorrhea among distance runners and other athletes been formally described (see Table 1). Feicht, Johnson, Martin, Sparks, and Wagner (1978) surveyed 400 women from the top 25 teams at the 1977 National Cross-Country Championships. One hundred sixty-two questionnaires were returned but after eliminating surveys due to incomplete response or use of birth control pills within 6 months preceding the study, the final sample consisted of 128 women. Athletes who had experienced three or fewer periods per year were classified as having secondary amenorrhea; all other subjects were classified as "regular." The incidence of secondary amenorrhea was high, 24%. The following year, Wakat, Sweeney, and Rogol (1982) surveyed the participants in the 1978 National Cross-Country Championships. Half of the respondents reported having only one period within the preceding 3 months and 2.6% reported having no periods within the last 6 months. Dale, Gerlach, and Wilhite (1979) also found a high incidence of amenorrhea (zero to five menses per year) among women who had run the Avon International Women's Marathon ($n = 168$). These runners were divided into two groups: (a) runners, those who ran more than 30 miles per week, and (b) joggers, those who ran 5 to 30 miles per week. The frequency of amenorrhea was higher in the runners (24%) than in the joggers (14%).

Contradictory results have been found in three surveys of large populations of women runners (Lutter & Cushman, 1982; Shangold & Levine, 1982; Speroff & Redwine, 1980). In a survey of almost 900 women runners in Portland, Oregon (Speroff & Redwine, 1980), only 6% of the women developed secondary amenorrhea after they started running. The exact definition of amenorrhea was not provided and training averaged less than 20 miles per week. In the second large survey, Shangold and Levine (1982) distributed questionnaires to over 1,800 women who entered the 1979 New York Marathon. Amenorrhea was defined as having no more than one period in the last 10 months. Of the 270 women who had regular menstrual cycles before training only 1% became amenorrheic during training. A strict definition of amenorrhea was used by Lutter and Cushman (1982) in a study of 350 women who had run either the 1980 Boston Marathon or a 10 km race in Minneapolis. Amenorrhea was defined as having no menstrual cycles in the last year. Only 3.4% of the sample had amenorrhea by this definition.

A question arising from these studies was whether amenorrhea existed among athletes participating in all sports. Sanborn, Martin, and Wagner (1982) surveyed 237 runners, 197 swimmers, and 33 cyclists. The incidence of amenorrhea was higher in all three groups as compared to controls. Significantly higher levels ($p < 0.05$) existed among the runners (25.7%) than swimmers (12.3%) or cyclists (12.1%). A large sample of collegiate varsity teams was surveyed by Carlberg, Buckman, Peake, and Riedesel (1983b). Using a definition of no menstrual cycles in the previous 3 months or four or fewer periods per year, 12.1% (17 of 140) had secondary amenorrhea. Dancers not only experience secondary amenorrhea but also have a high incidence of primary amenorrhea. Frisch, Wyshak, and Vincent (1980) reported data on 89 young ballet dancers. Twenty of the dancers developed amenorrhea (no menses for at least 3 consecutive months), and 30% reported irregular menstrual cycles. Using the same definition, a high frequency of secondary amenorrhea (37%) was also reported by Cohen, Kim, May, and Ertel (1982) among professional ballet dancers.

Defining Amenorrhea

The fact that these studies vary in the frequency of amenorrhea reported may be related to the different definitions of amenorrhea, or differences in athletic populations surveyed. The following criteria are suggested for standard definitions:

Regularly Menstruating:
- 12 periods per year at intervals of 28 ± 5 days,
- duration of each menses being 3 to 7 days, and
- ovulatory cycle(s) with a normal luteal phase length.

Athletic Amenorrhea:
- three or fewer periods per year with no more than one period in the 6 months prior to the study,
- regular menstrual cycles established within 18 months following menarche,
- training began before amenorrhea developed,
- discontinued taking birth control pills for at least 6 months before amenorrhea developed,
- negative gynecologic amenorrhea screen: complete medical history, physical examination, and laboratory evaluation to eliminate other causes of secondary amenorrhea, for example, hyperprolactinemia, hyperandrogenism, pituitary tumor, ovarian failure, and pregnancy.

The last criteria for each category would pertain to experimental research versus survey studies.

Short Luteal Phase

The frequency of menstrual irregularities and amenorrhea in athletes has been obtained from menstrual cycle histories. Thus the identification of normal or regular cycles has been based on the occurence of menses and cycle length, not on an endocrine basis. Several studies (Bonen, Belcastro, Ling, & Simpson, 1981; Prior, Yuen, Clement, Bowie, & Thomas, 1982; Shangold, Freeman, Thysen, & Gatz, 1979) have found that athletes usually have a short luteal phase. In the study by Bonen et al. (1981), four teenage swimmers were compared to a teenage control group and a group of fertile adult women. Blood samples were collected daily throughout one complete menstrual cycle. The follicular phase and luteal phase lengths were determined from the peak value of luteinizing hormone. The swimmers had a very short luteal phase (4.5 days) relative to the two control groups (7.8 days for the teenage group and 13.4 days for the adult group; $p < 0.05$). Further, the failure of progesterone to rise in the luteal phase suggested that the swimmers experienced anovulatory menstrual cycles. Since, however, only one menstrual cycle was evaluated, the frequency of anovulatory menstrual cycles cannot be predicted. While the teenage control group had a shorter luteal phase than the adult controls, an endocrine profile indicated normal ovulatory cycles.

Shangold et al. (1979) followed a 30-year-old woman to study the effects of long distance running on the menstrual cycle. Menstrual cycles remained unaltered throughout the training program. However, the length of the luteal phase slowly decreased with an increase in running mileage ($p < 0.01$). Prior and associates (1982) observed luteal phase shortening in two women training for a marathon. Daily basal body temperatures were used to determine the length of the luteal phase. As training mileage increased, the length of the luteal phase decreased. In one runner the length of the luteal phase decreased from 12 to 8 days and evolved into anovulatory cycles. Once training decreased these changes were reversed.

Results from these studies indicate that menstrual cycles based only on menstrual histories could be classified erroneously. This suggests that the incidence of amenorrhea reported so far could be conservative and is certainly very conservative if menstrual irregularities are considered.

Etiology of Athletic Amenorrhea

The high frequency of athletic amenorrhea observed among runners and ballet dancers has provided insight into the possible mechanism(s). These athletes characteristically have low body weight and low percentage body fat (Frisch et al., 1980; Wilmore & Brown, 1974). Both activities involve strenuous training, emotional stress, and training at a young age often before menarche. All of these factors have been implicated in the etiology of athletic amenorrhea (Baker, 1981). The most popular theory has been related to low body weight or more specifically, low body fat, the ''fat hypothesis.''

Fat hypothesis

Frisch and associates at Harvard have advanced the hypothesis that a direct relationship exists between a critical amount of fat and the onset and maintenance of menstruation (Frisch, 1972; Frisch, 1974; Frisch & McArthur, 1974; Frisch & Revelle, 1970; Frisch & Revelle, 1971; Frische, Revelle, & Cook, 1973). The theory has been based on the observation that menarche occurs at a critical weight rather than a specific age (Frisch, 1974; Frisch & Revelle, 1970; Frisch & Revelle, 1971). Further arguments used by Frisch and her associates to support their hypothesis were: (a) puberty in rats was reached at a specific body weight rather than a critical age (Kennedy & Mitra, 1963), (b) the steady decrease in age at menarche in the past century has been attributed to reaching the critical weight at an earlier age due to better nutrition than in the past (Tanner, 1962; Wyshak & Frisch, 1982), (c) clinical observation of amenorrhea in patients with anorexia nervosa and in patients with simple weight loss, which was reversed upon regaining weight (Knuth, Hull, & Jacobs, 1977; McArthur, Johnson, Hourihan, & Alonso, 1976; Wentz, 1980), and (d) aromatization of androgens to estrogen occurs in adipose tissue providing an extragonadal source of estrogen (Yen & Jaffe, 1978).

Several criticisms (Reeves, 1979; Trussell, 1980) have been directed at this hypothesis. The major one arises from the manner in which percent body fat was estimated from a height-weight equation (Mellits & Cheek, 1970) rather than a direct measurement. The critical values predicted by Frisch and co-workers can be seriously questioned, but the fat hypothesis merits consideration.

Female athletes are an excellent test for the fat hypothesis, especially runners and ballet dancers. Competitive distance runners have body fat levels as low as 5.9% (Wilmore & Brown, 1974). Preliminary findings in surveys of athletes tended to support the critical weight theory. Speroff and Redwine (1980) found that menstrual irregularities and amenorrhea were most common in runners who weighed less than 115 pounds and who lost more than 10 pounds after beginning training. Shangold and Levine (1982) also found amenorrheic runners to be significantly lighter in body weight than regularly menstruating women (50 kg vs. 55 kg respectively, $p < 0.05$).

Data on ballet dancers further supports the fat hypothesis. Ballet students with primary and secondary amenorrhea were lower in body weight than the regularly menstruating ballet dancers, 43.5 kg, 44.9 kg, and 47.0 kg respectively (Frisch, Wyshak, & Vincent, 1980). Professional ballet dancers with secondary amenorrhea also weigh less than regularly menstruating ballet dancers (Cohen, Kim, May, & Ertel, 1982). While average body weights were not provided, amenorrheic professional ballet dancers weighed a significantly lower percentage of ideal weight than dancers without menstrual irregularities (84.3%, 88.6%, respectively, $p < 0.05$).

Low body weight is not always synonymous with low body fat, however. Many athletes may initially lose weight with training but weight will usually stabilize. However, body fat can continue to decrease resulting in an alteration of the lean mass to body fat ratio. Boyden, Pamenter, Grosso, Stanforth, Rotkis, and Wilmore (1982) found that women training for a marathon had a decrease in percent fat without a change in body weight. A complex relationship exists between exercise and body composition. Thus, weight and height are not accurate predictors of body composition for athletes.

Several studies have compared either predicted or measured percent body fat of amenorrheic and regularly menstruating athletes. Schwartz, Cumming, Riordan, Selye, Yen, and Rebar (1981) compared amenorrheic runners (no menses for at least 4 months preceding the study) to three groups: (a) regularly menstruating runners who ran 30 miles per week, (b) regularly menstruating runners who ran 5 to 30 miles per week, and (c) nonrunning controls. Mean percentage body fat and weight were significantly lower in the amenorrheic runners in comparison to the other groups ($p < 0.01$). Body fat was estimated from skinfold thicknesses and was 18.2% for the amenorrheic runners, approximately 23% for both groups of regularly menstruating runners and 27.4% for the controls. Baker, Mathur, Kirk, and Williamson (1981) studied 23 women runners and found that the average percent body fat as estimated from skinfold thickness was not statistically different between amenorrheic (14.1%), and regularly menstruating runners (17.7%). Wakat et al. (1982) also found no significant differences in mean weight or sum of skinfold thicknesses between amenorrheic and regularly menstruating runners.

Using the hydrostatic weighing method but estimated residual volumes, Calabrese et al. (1983) found no difference in percent body fat between dancers with and without menstrual irregularities. Opposite results were found by Carlberg, Buckman, Peake, and Riedesel (1983a) in a group of 42 female athletes. These athletes were selected from college varsity sports (track and field, swimming and diving, tennis, and volleyball), high school varsity track and field, and a general population of distance runners. Percent body fat was measured by the hydrostatic weighing technique using a helium dilution method to calculate residual volume. The amenorrheic athletes (no menses in the previous 3 months or four periods in the previous year) had a significantly lower percent body fat, 13.1%, than the regularly menstruating group, 16.3% ($p < 0.05$). However, there was a considerable amount of overlap between the two groups (see Figure 1).

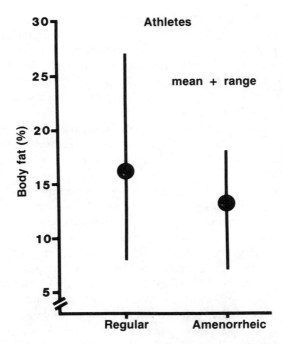

Figure 1.   Mean (± range) percent body fat of amenorrheic and regularly menstruating athletes. (After Carlberg et al., 1983a)

These results of the body fat studies are conflicting. However, the different methods used in determining body fat in the athletes, skinfold thickness versus hydrostatic weight, might contribute to the varied findings. Predicting body density from anthropometric variables such as skinfold measurements can result in large errors since the prediction equations are population specific (Jackson & Pollock, 1977). Hydrostatic weighing is one of the most accurate methods for measuring body density. However, actual measurement of the residual lung volume is crucial for computing body densities. Predicted values for residual volumes have a greater standard error than actual measured volumes, $\pm$ 500 ml, versus $\pm$ 100 ml respectively (Wilmore, 1969). For a 55 kg woman the estimation of body fat could have an error of $\pm$ 5% using a predicted residual volume versus $\pm$ 1% using an actual value.

The difficulty of understanding the relationship of body fat and body weight to athletic amenorrhea is further complicated by other variables. The following variables have appeared alone or in various combinations with the noted menstrual irregularities: late menarche, intense training prior to menarche, prior menstrual irregularities, intense training, nulliparity, young age, and psychological stress. Since these factors continually surface, each has been implicated with the onset of amenorrhea in athletes.

Late menarche

A later age of menarche has been reported for athletes than for nonathletes (Malina, Harper, Avent, & Campbell, 1973). The mean age of menarche was 13.6 years for 66 college track and field athletes and 12.2 years for 30 nonathletes, a significant difference. In a later study, Malina, Spirduso, Tate and Baylor (1978) reported that Olympic volleyball athletes have a significantly later age at menarche, 14.2 years when compared to high school and college athletes (13.0 years) and controls (12.3 years).

Ballet dancers with secondary amenorrhea also have delayed menarche. Menarche occurred at age 14 for two groups of amenorrheic ballet dancers (Calabrese et al., 1983; Frische et al., 1980) and at an even later age (15 years) in another study (Warren, 1980).

Among amenorrheic runners the findings have been diverse. Feicht et al. (1978) reported a significantly delayed menarche in amenorrheic middle-distance runners (14.1 years) versus a regularly menstruating group (13.3 years). A similar difference was reported by Wakat et al. (1982) between their amenorrheic (14.3 years) and regularly menstruating runners (12.9 years). Baker et al. (1981) also found that the age of menarche was significantly higher in amenorrheic runners (13.8 years) than in regularly menstruating runners (12.2 years). On the other hand, two studies on runners have found the age at menarche to be similar between the two groups (Schwartz et al., 1981; Shangold & Levine, 1982). Schwartz et al. (1981) reported a mean menarcheal age of 12.8 years for all the athletes and Shangold and Levine (1982) found menarche occurring at age 12.2 years for the amenorrheic runners and 12.7 years for the regularly menstruating runners.

The reason for the difference in these studies might be due to the age at which these athletes began training. The athletes who had a later menarche had begun their training at a very young age (Calabrese et al., 1983; Frisch et al., 1980) or around menarche (Wakat et al., 1982) while the women who began training in their mid-20s had menarcheal ages comparable to nonathletes (Schwartz et al., 1981; Shangold & Levine, 1982).

The cause of late menarche in some athletes is not known. Malina et al. (1978) raised an interesting question, does athletic training delay menarche, or do late maturers choose to be in certain sports? It has been suggested that for each year of training before menarche, the onset of menstruation will be delayed by 5 months (Frisch et al., 1981). Vandenbrouch, van Laar, and Valkenburg (1982) not only found that intense sports activity alone could delay menarche but that a synergistic effect occurred between sports participation and thinness in delaying menarche. How late menarche might be linked to athletic amenorrhea is not known.

Intense training prior to menarche

In only one study (Frisch et al., 1981) has the relationship of intense training prior to menarche and athletic amenorrhea been examined. The swimmers and runners who began training prior to menarche had 4 times the incidence of amenorrhea (no menses for 6 months) as those who began training after menarche.

Prior menstrual irregularities

Secondary amenorrhea has been reported to be more common in athletes who had a history of prior menstrual irregularities. Shangold and Levine (1982) stated that the single best predictor of amenorrhea in their sample of runners was prior menstrual irregularities. Schwartz et al. (1981) found that over 50% of their amenorrheic runners had past menstrual cycle irregularities.

Quantity of training

The frequency of amenorrhea has been positively correlated with the number of miles run per week (Feicht et al., 1978). The incidence steadily increased from 6% in those running less than 10 miles per week to 43% in those running more than 60 miles per week. In a later study, Sanborn et al. (1982) surveyed runners, cyclists, and swimmers to determine the incidence of amenorrhea in these endurance sports. Again weekly training mileage was correlated to the prevalence of amenorrhea among the runners; however, no such relationship could be shown for the swimmers and cyclists (see Figure 2). An association between training and frequency of menstrual dysfunction in dis-

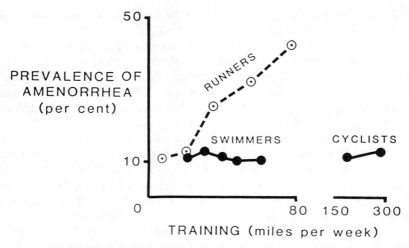

Figure 2. The prevalence of amenorrhea increased linearly as training mileage increased in runners ($p < 0.001$). Swimmers and cyclists had a 12% incidence regardless of training mileage. (Sanborn, Martin & Wagner, 1982)

tance runners was substantiated by Dale, Gerlach, and Wilhite (1979). In this study runners were divided into two groups: those who ran more than 30 miles per week (runners), and those who ran 5 to 30 miles per week (joggers). The controls ($n = 54$) experienced 4% amenorrhea (0 to 5 periods per year) in comparison to 24% of the joggers and 34% of the runners. Finally, support for an association was reported by Frisch et al. (1981) who found that the prevalence of amenorrhea in swimmers ($n = 21$) and runners ($n = 17$) increased during the training season in comparison to preseason.

Contradictory results have been reported by other investigators (Baker et al., 1981; Speroff & Redwine, 1980; Wakat, et al., 1982) who found no association between training mileage and the prevalence of amenorrhea. Disagreement is probably a result of study design. To investigate the correlation between prevalence of amenorrhea and training mileage the following criteria should be met: a large random sample, a wide range of training mileages, and dichotomous groups. In the latter criteria the groups should be divided into discrete mileages with equal number of data in each cell. In the Feicht et al. (1978) and Sanborn et al. (1982) studies, these criteria were met. In the Wakat et al. (1982) study, each point on the graph was selected based on an interval of 15 miles run per week. The number of athletes represented for each point is not known. Further, the range of weekly training mileage was from 20 to 80 and did not include the lower training mileages. Speroff and Redwine (1980) also found no correlation between weekly running mileage and amenorrhea. However, few of their women ran more than 20 miles per week. In the study by Baker et al. (1981) sample size was small ($n = 23$) and the groupings were not discrete.

All of these studies have examined quantity of training, miles per week, days per week, and months of training. None has examined the intensity of training, that is, at what percentage of maximum oxygen uptake do the athletes train. More work is required to determine whether certain characteristics of training cause athletic amenorrhea.

Hypothalamic maturity

Dale, Gerlach, and Wilhite (1979) were the first to note that prior pregnancy appeared to protect an athlete from developing amenorrhea. Their suggestion was based on the finding that prior pregnancy appeared to be inversely related to amenorrhea. Fifty percent of the runners who had never borne children (nulliparous) had menstrual irregularities while only 20% of the parous runners developed irregularities. The maturity of the hypothalamic-pituitary-ovarian system has also been related to the age of the athletes. In the previous study comparisons were not made between the ages of the amenorrheic and regularly menstruating runners or the ages of the nulliparous or parous runners. Baker et al. (1981) found that amenorrhea occurred more often in runners who were younger than 30 years of age (67%) than those 30 years of age or older (9%). Also, the nulliparous runners had a higher prevalence of amenorrhea than the parous runners; however, they were also younger. These findings suggest that younger nulliparous runners may be more susceptible to athletic amenorrhea because of an immature hypothalamic-pituitary-ovarian axis. These data support the observation of Erdelyi (1963) and Speroff and Redwine (1980) that younger women are more susceptible to menstrual dysfunction.

Psychological stress

An alternative explanation for athletic amenorrhea could be psychological stress stemming from intense training and competition. Amenorrheic middle-distance runners have subjectively rated the months they trained per year more intense than have the regularly menstruating group (Feicht et al., 1978). This finding was substantiated by Schwartz et al. (1981). Four psychological tests were also administered to the athletes to assess depression, anxiety, compulsive behavior, hypochondriac tendencies, and overall stress. No significant differences were found between the groups for any of the objective tests. However, the amenorrheic athletes subjectively evaluated more stress associated with running than the regularly menstruating group. According to the authors, the objective tests were not as sensitive as the subjective ratings in picking up subtle psychological differences.

Diet

There is evidence that nutritional status and diet can affect the reproductive system. While the mechanisms are unknown, poor dietary habits are often cited

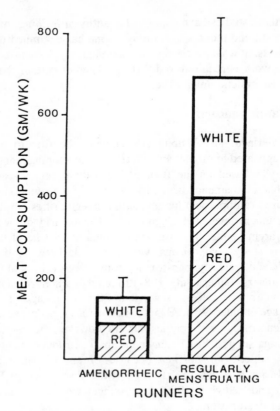

Figure 3.   Weekly total meat consumption, white meat (poultry and fish) and red meat, of amenorrheic and regularly menstruating runners. (Brooks et al., 1984)

as the explanation for amenorrhea in anorexia nervosa. A recent study by Brooks, Sanborn, Albrecht, and Wagner (1984) has examined the diets of amenorrheic ($n = 11$) and regularly menstruating runners ($n = 15$). The athletes kept dietary records for 7 consecutive days. The regularly menstruating runners ate five times more meat than the amenorrheic group ($p < 0.05$; see Figure 3). Vegetarianism was defined as consuming less than 200 gm/wk of meat (any combination of red or white). With this classification, 82% of the amenorrheic runners were considered vegetarian. Whether a diet high in plants or conversely low in meat plays a role in amenorrhea remains uncertain.

Hormonal alterations

The interrelationship within the hypothalamic-pituitary-ovarian axis is responsible for the events that lead to a normal menstrual cycle. The sole purpose of this cycle is the development of the ovum for fertilization: the ovarian cycle. Disruption of any part of the intricate negative and positive feed-back system of this axis can lead to menstrual dysfunction. Exercise-induced changes in endocrine hormones have been implicated in the etiology of athletic amenorrhea. The hormonal responses to exercise can be examined in two ways: by acute hormonal responses after a short bout of exercise, and chronic responses to long-term exercise. An in-depth review of the literature concerning hormonal alterations in females has been written by Loucks and Horvath (1984).

Acute hormonal response. Briefly, the effect of exercise on gonadotropins (follicular stimulating hormone, and luteinizing hormone) and steroid hormones (estrogen and progesterone) is difficult to interpret. Problems may stem from the fact that hormonal changes could reflect an increased production, hemoconcentration resulting from shifts in plasma volume during exercise, or a decreased clearance of the hormone in the blood (Cumming & Rebar, 1983). However, short-term exercise usually causes a rise in testosterone (Cumming & Rebar, 1983; Dale, Gerlach, Martin, & Alexander, 1979; Shangold, Gatz, & Thysen, 1981) and prolactin (Shangold, et al., 1979; Shangold et al., 1981). Increased levels of testosterone can cause feedback inhibition of luteinizing hormone secretion, thus resulting in menstrual dysfunction. The reason why elevated prolactin levels may cause amenorrhea is not clear. Prolactin may interfere with the responses between the hypothalamus and pituitary as well as the pituitary and ovaries.

Chronic hormonal response. Dale, Gerlach, and Wilhite (1979) showed in amenorrheic distance runners that luteinizing hormone and follicular-stimulating hormone levels were noncyclic and the values were consistently in the low to low-normal range. In comparison to a normal ovulatory cycle (see Figure 4), the values of serum estradiol and progesterone were always suppressed and showed no cyclic changes (see Figure 5). Serum testosterone

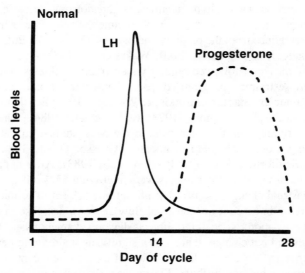

Figure 4.   Hormonal profile of a normal ovulatory nonrunner control. (Dale et al., 1979)

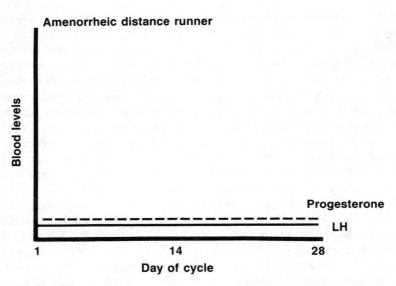

Amenorrheic distance runner

Figure 5.   Hormonal profile of an amenorrheic runner with an anovulatory cycle. (Dale et al., 1979)

levels were within the normal range but the mean for the runners was significantly higher than the mean for the controls. Because of the low and noncyclic nature of the gonadotropin secretion, it was concluded that the most probable site of the dysfunction was at the level of the pituitary or hypothalamus.

Preliminary findings suggest that the pituitary is functioning and that the site of dysfunction is at the hypothalamus. A gonadotropin-releasing hormone (GnRH) stimulation test in a small sample of amenorrheic athletes has resulted in normal secretions from the pituitary and ovaries. (McArthur, Bullen, Beitins, Pagano, Badger, & Klibanski, 1980; Wakat et al., 1982).

Two studies have followed regularly menstruating athletes as they undergo an exercise training program (Boyden, Pamenter, Grosso, et al., 1982; Boyden, Pamenter, Stanforth, Rotkis, & Wilmore, 1982; Boyden, Pamenter, Stanforth, Rotkis, & Wilmore, 1983; Bullen et al., 1984). The effect of endurance training on the menstrual cycle was studied in 19 regularly menstruating women (Boyden, Pamenter, Grosso, et al., 1982; Boyden, Pamenter, Stanforth et al., 1982; Boyden et al., 1983). After approximately 13.5 months of training, the subjects were averaging 63.4 miles running per week. Menstrual changes occurred in all but one subject. The major change was a decrease in amount of menstrual flow and/or a decrease in number of days of menstruation. None of the subjects developed amenorrhea. While total body weight did not change, there was a significant decrease in percent body fat from 25% to 22%. With the exclusion of estrodiol concentrations, in all of the hormones measured (thyroid hormones, thyroid-stimulating hormone, prolactin, and estrone/estrodiol ratio), the small changes that were observed were of questionable physiological importance.

Bullen and coworkers (1984) followed seven regularly menstruating women through an 8-week training program. The training regime did result in an increase in mean aerobic capacity; however, no significant changes occurred in the length and flow of the menstrual cycles or in plasma reproductive hormone levels (luteinizing hormone, follicular-stimulating hormone, and estradiol). Only β-endorphin + β-lipotropin and cortisol exhibited an increment as training progressed. However, ovarian function was disturbed as indicated by a decreased excretion of estriol, free progesterone, or both in four of the seven subjects. Within acute bouts of exercise, plasma concentrations of luteinizing hormone, follicular-stimulating hormone, and estradiol did not change while plasma concentrations of all antireproductive hormones (melatonin, prolactin, β-endorphin + β-lipotropin and cortisol) rose significantly.

Acute exercise and chronic exercise result in complex hormonal responses. More carefully controlled studies are needed to determine how exercise-induced changes in endocrine status cause the inappropriate feedback to the hypothalamus.

Multiple factors

The etiology of athletic amenorrhea remains unclear. In every study many variables have been associated with the menstrual irregularity. The failure to isolate one single factor has led to the multifactor theory: a combination of associated factors synergistically result in reproductive dysfunction. Two studies have done multiple regression analysis on the various factors associated with athletic amenorrhea (Galle, Freeman, Galle, Huggins, & Sondheimer, 1983; Gray & Dale, 1983). The purposes of the studies were to determine which combination of factors could predict menstrual status. In the study by Gray and Dale (1983) a model was presented that proposed a linkage between training variables, percent body fat, age, and the number of menstrual cycles per year.

Both studies were able to account for approximately 30% of the menstrual status variability. A large percentage of the variance has not been explained. However, athletic amenorrhea is a complex issue, the variables are not discrete but are complexly related. These findings do not rule out the possibility that each individual athlete may have her own combination of various factors that results in amenorrhea.

Is Athletic Amenorrhea Adaptive?

Does athletic amenorrhea effect performance? Elite endurance athletes have low ventilatory responses to lower than normal amounts of oxygen (hypoxia) and higher than normal amounts of carbon dioxide (Byrne-Quinn, Weil, Sodal, Filley, & Grover, 1971; Martin, Sparks, Zwillich, & Weil, 1979). The reason for this association is not clear; however, if low respiratory drives are advantageous to exercise performance, perhaps by lowering ventilatory work, any factor that increases ventilation past the minimal amount necessary could adversely affect athletic performance. Progesterone is a potent ventilatory stimulant (Pernoll, Metcalfe, Kovack, Wachel, & Dunham, 1975; Zwillich, Natalino, Sutton, & Weil, 1978). Male distance runners reduced performance when given progesterone (Martin, Weil, Zwillich, & Grover, 1978). Therefore, the low and noncyclic levels of progesterone in females with athletic amenorrhea may enhance performance. Schoene, Robertson, Pierson, and Peterson (1981) investigated the role of progesterone in exercise performance and ventilatory responses. Three groups of females were tested: (a) six regularly menstruating nonathletes, (b) six regularly menstruating athletes, and (c) six amenorrheic athletes. The respiratory test was made by determining the ventilatory response to hypoxia (expressed as the hyperbolic shape parameter, A; the higher the A, the more vigorous is the ventilatory response to hypoxia). When progesterone is present during the luteal phase in nonathletes, A is high, as expected (see Table 2). In menstruating, highly trained athletes, A is lower than controls, but still changes during the menstrual cycle. Ventilatory drives and exercise ventilation were increased during the luteal phase for both athletes and controls, but exercise performance was only decreased among the controls, not the athletes. In contrast to expectations, in highly trained amenorrheic athletes, A is not lower than in highly trained menstruating runners. These data provide evidence that lack of progesterone in the amenorrheic athletes confers no ventilatory advantage as measured by either hypoxic or hypercapnic ventilatory drives.

Table 2 Hypoxic ventilatory response as expressed by shape parameter A (Mean ± SEM).

Athlete	N	Follicular	Luteal	Probability
Menstruating nonathletes	6	102.2 ±32.7	203.8 ±16.1	<0.02
Menstruating athletes	6	81.7 ±16.9	104.6 ±9.7	<0.05
Amenorrheic athletes	6	108.6 ±36.4	110.7 ±30.9	NS

Reversibility

Two questions of utmost importance to the female athlete are whether athletic amenorrhea is irreversible and if return of menses is associated with a normal fertility. The current literature contains only a few studies dealing with this important issue. Preliminary evidence from a survey of distance runners (Stager, Ritchie-Flanagan, & Robertshaw, 1984) and a case study (Prior et al., 1982) indicate that once training is reduced normal menstrual cycles will resume. Of the surveyed runners who had menstrual irregularities associated with training, menstrual cycles returned in an average of 2 months after discontinuation of training (Stager et al., 1984). Many questions are unanswered concerning this important area: Is the reversibility of athletic amenorrhea universal? Are the athletes fertile after they reduce training? Do regular menses last over a period of years? What is the mechanism behind resumption of menses?

Harmful Effects

If it is true that normal menses will resume once training is reduced, then there would not appear to be any harmful effects on the reproductive system from athletic amenorrhea. But there may be a potentially deleterious effect on the skeletons of these athletes. A preliminary report concerning this issue was made by Cann, Martin, Genant, and Jaffe (1984). A Computed Tomography scanner was used to study the spinal bone density of amenorrheic women (a subgroup of hypothalamic amenorrheic subjects also exercised) and found the density to be below normal. Normally, bone under mechanical stress has increased density (Aloia, Cohn, Ostuni, Cane, & Ellis, 1981). Thus, it was unexpected that bone mineral content would be reduced in the amenorrheic subgroup who exercised. One explanation could be that amenorrheic athletes have low estrogen levels. Low estrogen states are associated with a reduction in bone mass and low bone mass has been documented in postmenopausal women who normally experience a drop in estrogen (Lindsay et al., 1978).

The relationship between athletic amenorrhea and bone mass was examined by Linell, Stager, Blue, Oyster and Robertshaw, (1984). Three groups of women were compared: amenorrheic runners, regularly menstruating runners, and regularly menstruating sedentary controls. Bone mineral content was measured at two sites on the radius using a single-photon densitometer. No significant differences were found for either radial bone mineral content measurement between the groups. Also, the average of the bone mineral content for all groups was within normal values.

Measurements of the radius using a single-photon absorptiometer are correlated to the skeletal bone mass and are reliable. However, the measurements of the lumbar spine using a dual-photon absorptiometer are more sensitive to bone mass changes (Lindberg et al., 1984). To date, two studies have examined both the bone masses in the radius and the lumbar spine in amenorrheic athletes.

Drinkwater et al. (1984) compared the bone mass of 14 amenorrheic athletes (no more than 1 period in the previous 12 months) to 14 regularly menstruating athletes to determine whether skeletal mass is compromised by a hypoestrogenic status. The two groups of athletes were matched for age, height, weight, sport, and frequency and duration of daily training. Single-photon and dual-photon absorptiometry were used to measure regional bone mass at the distal radius and lumbar vertebrae, respectively. Bone mineral density at the radius did not differ between groups; however, the mineral density of the lumbar vertebrae was significantly lower in the amenorrheic group of athletes compared to the regularly menstruating athletes ($p < 0.01$).

Similar results were found by Lindberg and co-workers (1984). Subjects were grouped according to their menstrual history and training status: (a) amenorrheic runners, no periods for the previous 6 months; (b) oligomenorrheic runners, menses occurred every 6 weeks to 6 months; (c) regularly menstruating runners, (d) regularly menstruating sedentary controls, and (e) postmenopausal women. Radial bone mass was determined by single-photon absorptiometry in all subjects and spinal bone mineral measurements were determined in 8 of the 11 amenorrheic runners with a dual-photon absorptiometer. The amenorrheic runners had a significantly lower bone mass in both radial sites in comparison to the regularly menstruating runners and controls. Further, the average lumbar spinal bone mineral content was less than normal in the amenorrheic runners.

Many questions remain unanswered regarding skeletal integrity of amenorrheic athletes. These findings should not be interpreted that female athletes should cease training. However, an awareness is needed among physicians and athletes that some amenorrheic athletes may have a decrease in bone density.

Summary

Secondary amenorrhea is common among athletes and can be as high as 45% among long distance runners. However, there is a large variation in incidence rates between studies which stems in part from the lack of a consistent definition of amenorrhea. Several studies have defined amenorrhea as having no menses for at least 3 consecutive months to one study which used the definition of having no periods in the past year. These values have been obtained from population surveys in which determination of regularity has been based solely on the length of the cycle and not on endocrine data. Short luteal phases have been observed in some athletes who were originally classified as regularly menstruating. An erroneous classification could result based on menstrual histories alone. These findings suggest that, if anything, the incidence of amenorrhea reported is underestimated.

Since distance runners and ballet dancers have the highest frequencies of amenorrhea and are characteristically low in body weight and body fat, a "fat hypothesis" has evolved. Two major lines of evidence have been used as support for the fat hypothesis: menarche occurs at a critical weight, and some anorexia nervosa patients begin menstruating after regaining weight. Body weights of amenorrheic athletes are less than those with regular menstrual cycles. However, findings on percent body fat have been conflicting. There could be two reasons. First, percent body fat has been calculated from two different methods, skinfold thickness measurements and hydrostatic weighing. In the latter measurement, additional error could result from using predicted versus actual measured residual volume. Second, multiple factors have existed in every study. These factors are late menarche, intense training prior to menarche, prior menstrual irregularities, intense training, nulliparity, young age, psychological stress, hormonal imbalance, and diet. These variables alone or in various combinations have been implicated in the development of athletic amenorrhea. At this time there is no clear explanation for the etiology of athletic amenorrhea.

References

Aloia, J.F., Cohn, S.H., Ostuni, J.A., Cane, R., & Ellis, K. (1978). Prevention of involutional bone loss by exercise. *Annuals of Internal Medicine, 89*, 356-358.

Baker, E.R. (1981). Menstrual dysfunction and hormonal status in athletic women: A review. *Fertility and Sterility, 36*, 691-696.

Baker, E.R., Mathur, R.S., Kirk, R.F., & Williamson, H.O. (1981). Female runners and secondary amenorrhea: Correlation with age, parity, mileage, and plasma hormonal and sex-hormone-binding globulin concentrations. *Fertility and Sterility, 36*, 183-187.

Bausenwien, I. (1954). Zur frage sport und menstruation. *Deutsche Medizinische Wochenschrift, 79*, 1526-32.

Bonen, A., Belcastro, A.N., Ling, W.Y., & Simpson, A.A. (1981). Profiles of selected hormones during menstrual cycles of teenage athletes. *Journal of Applied Physiology, 50*, 545-551.

Boyden, T.W., Pamenter, R.W., Grosso, D., Stanforth, P., Rotkis, T., & Wilmore, J.H. (1982). Prolactin responses, menstrual cycles, and body composition of women runners. *Journal of Clinical Endocrinology and Metabolism, 54*, 711-714.

Boyden, T.W., Pamenter, R.W., Stanforth, P., Rotkis, T., & Wilmore, J.H. (1982). Evidence for mild thyroidal impairment in women undergoing endurance training. *Journal of Clinical Endocrinology and Metabolism, 53*, 53-56.

Boyden, T.W., Pamenter, R.W., Stanforth, P., Rotkis, T., & Wilmore, J.H. (1983). Sex steroids and endurance running in women. *Fertility and Sterility, 39*, 629-632.

Brooks, S.M., Sanborn, C.F., Albrecht, B.H., & Wagner, W.W., Jr. (1984). Diet in athletic amenorrhea. *Lancet, 1*(8376), 559-560.

Bullen, B.A., Skrinar, G.S., Beitins, I.Z., Carr, D.B., Reppert, S.M., Dotson, C.O., Fencl, M. de M., Gervino, E.V., & McArthur, J.W. (1984). Endurance training effects on plasma hormonal responsiveness and sex hormone secretion. *Journal of Applied Physiology, 56*, 1453-1463.

Byrne-Quinn, E., Weil, J.V., Sodal, I.E., Filley, G.F., & Grover, R.F. (1971). Ventilatory control in athletes. *Journal of Applied Physiology, 30*, 91-98.

Calabrese, L.H., Kirkendall, D.T., Floyd, M., Rapoport, S., Williams, G.W., Weiker, G.G., & Bergfeld, J.A. (1983). Menstrual abnormalities, nutritional patterns and body composition in female classical ballet dancers. *The Physician and Sportsmedicine, 11*, 86-98.

Cann, C.E., Martin, M.C., Genant, H.K., & Jaffe, R.B. (1984). Decreased spinal mineral content in amenorrheic women. *Journal of the American Medical Association, 5*, 626-629.

Carlberg, K.A., Buckman, M.T., Peake, G.T., & Riedesel, M.L. (1983a). Body composition of oligo/amenorrheic athletes. *Medicine and Science in Sports and Exercise, 15*, 215-217.

Carlberg, K.S., Buckman, M.T., Peake, G.T., & Riedesel, M.L. (1983b). A survey of menstrual function in athletes. *European Journal of Applied Physiology, 51*, 211-212.

Cohen, J.L., Kim, C.S., May, P.B., & Ertel, N.H. (1982). Exercise, body weight, and professional ballet dancers. *The Physician and Sportsmedicine, 10*, 92-101.

Cumming, D.C., & Rebar, R.W. (1983). Exercise and reproductive function in women. *American Journal of Industrial Medicine, 4*, 113-125.

Dale, E., Gerlach, D.H., Martin, D.E., & Alexander, C.R. (1979). Physical fitness profiles and reproductive physiology of the female distance runner. *The Physician and Sportsmedicine, 7*, 83-95.

Dale, E., Gerlach, D.H., & Wilhite, A.L. (1979). Menstrual dysfunction in distance runners. *Obstetrics and Gynecology, 54*, 47-53.

Drew, F. (1961). Epidemiology of secondary amenorrhea. *Journal of Chronic Diseases, 14*, 396-406.

Drinkwater, B.L., Nilson, K., Chesnut, C.H., Bremner, W.J., Shainholtz, S., & Southworth, M.B. (1984). Bone mineral content of amenorrheic and eumenorrheic athletes. *New England Journal of Medicine, 311*, 277-281.

Erdelyi, G.J. (1963). Gynecological survey of female athletes. *Journal of Sports Medicine and Physical Fitness,* **2,** 174-179.

Feicht, C.B., Johnson, T.S., Martin, B.J., Sparks, K.E., & Wagner, W.W., Jr. (1978). Secondary amenorrhea in athletes. *Lancet,* **2,** 1145-1146.

Fries, H., Nillius, S.J., & Pettersson, F. (1974). Epidemiology of secondary amenorrhea. *American Journal of Obstetrics and Gynecology,* **118,** 473-479.

Frisch, R.E. (1972). Weight at menarche: Similarity for well-nourished and undernourished girls at differing ages and evidence for historical constancy. *Pediatrics,* **50,** 445-450.

Frisch, R.E. (1974). A method of prediction of age of menarche from height and weight at ages 9 through 13 years. *Pediatrics,* **53,** 384-390.

Frisch, R.E., Gotz-Welbergen, A.V., McArthur, J.W., Albright, T., Witschi, J., Bullen, B., Birnholz, J., Reed, R.B., & Herman, H. (1981). Delayed menarche and amenorrhea of college athletes in relation to age of onset of training. *Journal of the American Medical Association,* **246,** 1559-1563.

Frisch, R.E., & McArthur, J.W. (1974). Menstrual cycles: Fatness as a determinant of minimum weight for height necessary for their maintenance or onset. *Science,* **185,** 949-951.

Frisch, R.E., & Revelle, R. (1970). Height and weight at menarche and a hypothesis of critical body weights and adolescent events. *Science,* **169,** 397-399.

Frisch, R.E., & Revelle, R. (1971). The height and weight of girls and boys at the time of initiation of the adolescent growth spurt in height and weight and the relationship to menarche. *Human Biology,* **43,** 140-159.

Frisch, R.E., Revelle, R., & Cook, S. (1973). Components of weight at menarche and the initiation of the adolescent growth spurt in girls: Estimated total water, lean body weight and fat. *Human Biology,* **45,** 469-483.

Frisch, R.E., Wyshak, G., & Vincent, L. (1980). Delayed menarche and amenorrhea in ballet dancers. *New England Journal of Medicine,* **303,** 17-19.

Galle, P.C., Freeman, E.W., Galle, M.G., Huggins, G.R., & Sondheimer, S.T. (1983) Physiologic and psychologic profiles in a survey of women runners. *Fertility and Sterility,* **39,** 633-639.

Gray, D.P., & Dale, E. (1983). Variables associated with secondary amenorrhea in women runners. *Journal of Sports Sciences,* **1,** 55-67.

Jackson, A.S., & Pollock, M.L. (1977). Prediction accuracy of body density, lean body weight, and total body volume equations. *Medicine and Science in Sports,* **9,** 197-210.

Kennedy, G.G., & Mitra, J. (1963). Body weight and food intake as indicating factors for puberty in the rat. *Journal of Physiology* (London), **166,** 408-418.

Knuth, U.A., Hull, M.G.R., & Jacobs, H.S. (1977). Amenorrhea and loss of weight. *British Journal of Obstetrics and Gynecology,* **84,** 801-807.

Lindberg, J.S., Fears, W.B., Hunt, M.M., Powell, M.R., Boll, D., & Wade, C.E. (1984). Exercise-induced amenorrhea and bone density. *Annals of Internal Medicine*, **101**, 647-648.

Lindsay, R., Hart, D.M., MacLean, A., Clark, A.C., Kraszewski, A., & Garwood, J. (1978). Bone response to termination of oestrogen treatment. *Lancet*, **1** (2), 1325-1327.

Linnell, S.L., Stager, J.M., Blue, P.W., Oyster, N., & Robertshaw, D. (1984). Bone mineral content and menstrual regularity in female runners. *Medicine and Science in Sports and Exercise*, **4**,343-348.

Loucks, A.B., & Horvath, S.M. (1985). Athletic amenorrhea: A review. *Medicine and Science in Sports and Exercise*, **17**, 56-72.

Lutter, J.M., & Cushman, S. (1982). Menstrual patterns in female runners. *The Physician and Sportsmedicine*, **10**, 60-72.

Malina, R.M., Harper, A.B., Avent, H.H., & Campbell, D.E. (1973). Age at menarche in athletes and non-athletes. *Medicine and Science in Sports*, **5**, 11-13.

Malina, R.M., Spirduso, W.W., Tate, C., & Baylor, A.M. (1978). Age at menarche and selected menstrual characteristics in athletes at different levels and in different sports. *Medicine and Science in Sports*, **10**, 218-222.

Martin, B.M., Sparks, K.E., Zwillich, C.W., & Weil, J.V. (1979). Low exercise ventilation in endurance athletes. *Medicine and Science in Sports*, **11**, 181-185.

Martin, B.J., Weil, J.V., Zwillich, C.W., & Grover, R.F. (1978). Drugs that alter the ventilatory response to hypoxia alter exercise ventilation. *Federation Proceedings*, **37**, 429. (Abstract)

McArthur, J.W., Bullen, B.A., Beitins, I.Z., Pagano, M., Badger, T.M., & Klibanski, A. (1980). Hypothalamic amenorrhea in runners of normal body composition. *Endocr. Res. Commun.*, **7**, 89-91.

McArthur, J.W., Johnson, L., Hourihan, J., & Alonso, C. (1976). Endocrine studies during the refeeding of young women with nutritional amenorrhea and infertility. *Mayo Clinic Proceedings*, **51**, 607-616.

Mellits, E.B. & Cheek, D.B. (1970). The assessment of body water and fatness from infancy to adulthood. *Monograph for Society Research in Child Development*, **35**, 12-26.

Pernoll, M.L., Metcalfe, J., Kovack, P.A., Wachel, R., & Durham, M.J. (1975). Ventilation during rest and exercise in pregnancy and post-partum. *Respiratory Physiology*, **25**, 295-310.

Prior, J.C., Yuen, B.H., Clement, P., Bowie, L., & Thomas, J. (1982). Reversible luteal phase changes and infertility associated with marathon training. *Lancet*, **2**, 269-270.

Reeves, J. (1979). Estimating fatness. *Science*, **204**, 881.

Sanborn, C.F., Martin, B.J., & Wagner, W.W., Jr. (1982). Is athletic amenorrhea specific to runners? *American Journal of Obstetrics and Gynecology, 143*, 859-861.

Schoene, R.B., Robertson, H.T., Pierson, D.J., & Peterson, A.P. (1981). Respiratory drives and exercise in menstrual cycles of athletic and non-athletic women. *Journal of Applied Physiology, 50*, 1300-1305.

Schwartz, B., Cumming, D.C., Riordan, E., Selye, M., Yen, S.S.C., & Rebar, R.W. (1981). Exercise-associated amenorrhea: A distinct entity? *American Journal of Obstetrics and Gynecology, 141*, 662-670.

Shangold, M.M., Freeman, R., Thysen, B., & Gatz, M. (1979). The relationship between long-distance running, plasma progesterone, and luteal phase length. *Fertility and Sterility, 31*, 130-133.

Shangold, M.M., Gatz, M.L., & Thysen, B. (1981). Acute effects of exercise on plasma concentrations of prolactin and testosterone in recreational women runners. *Fertility and Sterility, 35*, 699-702.

Shangold, M.M., & Levine, H.S. (1982). The effect of marathon training upon menstrual function. *American Journal of Obstetrics and Gynecology, 143*, 862-869.

Speroff, L., & Redwine, D.B. (1980). Exercise and menstrual function. *The Physician and Sportsmedicine, 8*, 42-52.

Stager, J.M., Ritchie-Flanagan, B., & Robertshaw, D. (1984). Reversibility of amenorrhea in athletes. *New England Journal of Medicine, 310*, 51-52.

Tanner, J.M. (1962). *Growth at adolescence* (2nd ed.). Oxford: Blackwell Scientific Publications.

Trussell, J. (1980). Statistical flaws in evidence for the Frisch hypothesis that fatness triggers menarche. *Human Biology, 52*, 711-720.

Vandenbroucke, J.P., van Laar, A., & Valkenburg, H.A. (1982). Synergy between thinness and intensive sports activity in delaying menarche. *British Medical Journal, 284*, 1907-1908.

Wakat, D.K., Sweeney, K.A., & Rogol, A.D. (1982). Reproductive system function in women cross-country runners. *Medicine and Science in Sports and Exercise, 14*, 263-269.

Warren, M.P. (1980). The effect of exercise on pubertal progression and reproductive function in girls. *Journal Clinical Endocrinology and Metabolism, 51*, 1150-1156.

Wentz, A. (1980). Body weight and amenorrhea. *Obstetrics and Gynecology, 56*, 482-487.

Wilmore, J. (1969). The use of actual, predicted and constant residual volumes in the assessment of body composition by underwater weighing. *Medicine and Science in Sports, 1*, 87-89.

Wilmore, J.H., & Brown, C. (1974). Physiological profiles of women distance runners. *Medicine and Science in Sports, 6*, 178-181.

Wyshak, G., & Frisch, R.E. (1982). Evidence for secular trend in age of menarche. *New England Journal of Medicine, 306*, 1033-1035.

Yen, S.C., & Jaffe, R.B. (1978). *Reproductive endocrinology.* Philadelphia: W.B. Saunders.

Zwillich, C.W., Natalino, M.R., Sutton, F.D., & Weil, J.V. (1978). Effect of progesterone on chemosensitivity in normal men. *Journal of Laboratory Clinical Medicine, 92*, 262-269.

9 Injuries in Female Distance Runners

Karen L. Nilson
University of Washington

The percentage of the population that jogs or runs has increased exponentially over the last decade, and the increase in the number of women participating in running has been especially noticeable. With this increase in the popularity of running has come an increased awareness of a variety of injuries that arise from participation in sports requiring repetitive movements. These injuries to the musculoskeletal system are referred to as overuse injuries. They take a variety of forms and may affect many anatomical sites, but they share a common etiology: repetitive stress on certain anatomical structures that leads to injury. While no overuse injuries are unique to women, differences have been observed in injury rates between men and women for specific injuries and certain classifications of injuries. The purpose of this chapter is to explore the extent of the problem of overuse injuries associated with running, classify and discuss the etiology and mechanisms of these injuries, and explore some differences between men and women with respect to specific injuries.

Extent of the Problem

Pagliano and Jackson (1980) have pointed out a low incidence of disabling injuries in distance runners, but they found "strong potential for chronic overuse syndromes." The overall incidence of injury in runners is not well documented, but a *Runner's World* article in 1977 estimated that two out of three of its readers would have an injury significant enough to cause them to stop or cut back on running or see a doctor within the following year (Henderson, 1977). Also, more than one third of the injuries seen at a metropolitan sports clinic between 1975 and 1979 were related to running or jogging (Witman, Melvin, & Nicholas, 1981). Even when only one area of the anatomy—the knee—is considered, estimates of injury rates range from 23% to 50% (Newell & Bramwell, 1984).

The extent of the problem for women runners is poorly documented. Most studies of runners' injuries report fewer female than male patients. For example,

149

James, Bates, and Ostering (1978) reported only 16% of their 232 patients were female, and Pagliano and Jackson (1980) reported on injuries in 330 female and 747 male runners (31% females) treated over a 10-month period. However, there is no indication of the percentage of women in the running population from which the authors drew their cases.

A retrospective survey of clinical records done by Clement, Taunton, Smart, and McNicol (1981) provides some information regarding differences in injury rates between men and women. In their study, 1,819 injuries were identified in 1,650 runners between 1978 and 1980. To estimate the relative numbers of males and females and the age distribution of the running population from which they were drawing their patients, the authors surveyed the participants in a local fun run. Nearly 60% of the patients in their study were men, but the authors concluded that women under 30 years of age were at greatest risk of developing overuse injuries from running. They based this conclusion on the fact that 49% of their patients under 30 were female, while only 36% of the fun run participants under 30 were female. Of the fun run participants over 30, 23.5% were women, while 28% of the patients in the same age-group were women.

Even less information is available on elite female distance runners. It might be expected that elite female athletes would have a lower predisposition to musculoskeletal injury than average females to enable them to withstand the extensive training necessary to achieve world class times over long distances. But, perhaps because of their extensive training, even the group of runners who qualified for the first U.S. Women's Olympic Marathon Trials had a relatively high incidence of injuries. Ninety-three (44%) out of 210 who completed medical history questionnaires reported a history of musculoskeletal problems that they considered significant. Twenty-nine of the 267 qualifiers were unable to compete in the trials because of injury, and the performance of many others was hampered by injury.

It can be concluded that the incidence of injuries in runners is relatively high. Although the severity of these injuries is usually minor, they tend to be chronic and recurring. Problems are seen in both males and females, and inexperienced as well as elite-class runners are at risk.

Etiology

The vast majority of injuries that occur in running are overuse injuries, which take the form of stress fractures or inflammatory processes such as tendinitis or bursitis. These conditions are the result of "repetitive forces on a structure beyond the abilities of that specific structure to withstand such a force" (Stanish, 1984). The causes of overuse injuries can be divided into extrinsic and intrinsic (anatomical) factors. James et al. (1978) estimated that 60% of the injuries in their series were secondary to extrinsic factors classified as training errors. The most common problem, accounting for 29% of the training errors, was excessive mileage. Other errors in training include rapid increases in various components of the training schedule; the addition of interval training to increase speed; increased hills; bounding or jumping exercises; increased time on hard surfaces; and slanted surfaces such as a beach or the shoulder of a road.

Running shoes are another external factor that contributes to a high percentage of injuries. Shoe technology has increased greatly over the last decade. Specific features included in many models of shoes such as air cushions, medial wedges, added rear foot support and the like can be of tremendous benefit to an individual runner. Some of these features can, however, merely exacerbate existing anatomical or training problems if the shoes and the special features are improperly chosen for a given runner. Also, excessive wear on a pair of shoes can lead to injury. Common shoe problems found by Clement et al. (1981) included inadequate heel wedging, soft or loose heel counters, excessive lateral heel wear, narrow toe boxes, inflexible soles under the metatarsals, and improper application of sole repair material. A variety of intrinsic or anatomical factors contribute to overuse injuries associated with running (James et al., 1978; Clement et al., 1981). Each foot strikes the ground an estimated 400 to 1,000 times per mile at a force estimated by Brody (1980) to be three to eight times body weight. Much of that force is transmitted upward to other anatomical structures, so even minor abnormalities of no consequence in other sports may become significant factors in the development of injuries in running. Although many anatomical factors have been identified, both James et al. (1978) and Clement et al. (1981) placed great emphasis on foot alignment, especially excessive pronation, which occurred in 58% of James' series. Pronation, which occurs at the subtalar joint with associated motions of the lower extremity, "unlocks" the foot and allows for adaptation to the running surface. Because pronation is associated with other motions of the lower extremity, abnormalities in alignment or motion of other structures can cause excessive pronation. Many of the overuse problems common in running include chondromalacia (Buchbinder, Napora, & Biggs, 1979), stress fractures (Taunton, Clement, & Webber, 1981), shinsplints (Lilletvedt, Kreighbaum, & Phillips, 1979; Viitasalo & Kvist, 1983), and Achilles tendinitis (Clement, Taunton, & Smart, 1984) have been associated with excessive pronation.

Leg-length discrepancy is another common finding often implicated in overuse problems for runners. After studying 35 male marathon runners, most of whom had a difference of less than 5mm, Gross (1983) concluded that minor discrepancies (less than 2.5 cm) "did not appear to have a deleterious effect on function in marathon runners, nor was the use of a lift demonstrated to be effective." His study, however, included only runners who had successfully completed a marathon, and there were only seven runners with discrepancies of greater than one cm. The study gave no indication how many runners with leg-length discrepancies may have been forced to stop or reduce training because of injuries.

Other intrinsic factors that predispose a runner to injury include abnormalities in muscle balance, strength, or flexibility. For instance, the
importance of the balance of pull between the vastus medialis on the medial
side of the patella and the vastus lateralis on the lateral side is widely recognized
(Henry & Crosland, 1979; Steadman, 1979; Levine, 1979; Wild, Franklin,
& Woods, 1982). Weakness of the vastus medialis combines with other
predisposing anatomical factors to cause abnormal tracking of the patella with
resultant patellofemoral pain, chondromalacia, or subluxation or dislocation
of the patella.

Lack of sufficient flexibility is a significant factor in many cases of
tendinitis. Iliotibial band friction syndrome, a common cause of knee pain in
runners (Noble, 1980; Sutker, Jackson, & Pagliano, 1981; Noble, Hajek, &
Porter, 1982; Lindenberg, Pinshaw, & Noakes, 1984), as well as Achilles tendinitis and peritendinitis (Smart, Taunton, & Clement, 1980), and plantar
fasciitis (Roy, 1983; Taunton, Clement, & McNicol, 1982) are associated with
tightness in their associated muscle groups or tendons.

Greater joint laxity is another characteristic thought to occur more
frequently in females. However, in a study investigating whether joint looseness is a trait or a function of a particular joint, the authors concluded that
"women may be looser than men on some tests, but the joint-looseness trait
is not sex related." (Marshall, Johanson, Wieckiewicz, Tischler, Koslin, Zeno,
& Meyers, 1980). As will be discussed later, women have been found to have
fewer Achilles tendon problems. Perhaps the difference is related to greater
flexibility in the posterior leg and thigh as evidenced by greater palm-to-floor
flexibility found by the same study to be one of the sex-related joint looseness
variables.

A variety of causes of overuse injuries have been discussed. The most
common problems leading to injury in runners are extrinsic errors in training
and are therefore not necessarily related to gender. Certain intrinsic anatomical
factors may relate to sex differences and lead to differences in injury patterns.
These patterns will be discussed later.

As pointed out by Wells and Plowman (1983), the frequency distribution
of most physical characteristics fall along a bell-shaped curve, and although
the means of the curves between men and women may be different, there is
often greater variation between two people of the same sex than between the
means of different sexes. This is true for some of the anatomical variations
that contribute to injury in runners, but some attributes are associated more
frequently with women and may help explain some of the differences in rates
of specific injuries between men and women.

The increased width of the female pelvis is often mentioned as a
contributing factor in overuse problems around the knee and hip. The Q-angle
(the angle formed by the intersection of a line drawn perpendicular from the
anterior superior iliac spine and a line from the tibial tubercle through the midpoint of the patella) is increased by widening the distance between the iliac
crests. The angle can also be increased by genu valgum (knock-knee deformity),

which also seems to occur more frequently in females. A Q-angle greater than 20° is considered abnormal and is believed to predispose to patellofemoral problems.

Classification of Injuries

As implied by the name, overuse syndromes share a common mechanism of injury: repeated submaximal stresses on a given structure that overwhelm its capacity to respond to the stress and repair itself. In most instances the injured tissue sets up an inflammatory response to the microtrauma that has occurred. This response leads to the clinical symptoms we recognize as heat, redness, swelling, and pain. A variety of tissues are susceptible to such injury.

Tendons are dense connective tissue composed of collagen fibers arranged in parallel with interspersed mucopolysaccharide. They are surrounded by either a loose aereolar connective tissue, the peritendon, as in the case of the Achilles tendon, or a true synovial sheath. In areas where a tendon may be exposed to pressure or wear, it is protected by either a synovial sheath or a bursa. Any of these structures may become inflamed, leading to tendinitis, tenosynovitis, peritendinitis, or bursitis. Another common site of inflammation is the insertion of tendon into bone. Most cases of posterior tibial tendinitis, which has been referred to as medial tibial stress syndrome or shinsplints (D'Ambrosia, Zelis, Chuinard, & Wilmore, 1977; Mubarek, Gould, Lee, Schmidt, & Hargens, 1982), fall into this category. Other connective tissue structures, such as the planter fascia (running from the calcaneous to the metatarsal heads), the peripatellar retinaculum (Fulkerson, 1982) and plica (synovial folds in the knee) (Hardaker, Whipple, & Bassett, 1980; Nottage, Sprague, Auerbach, & Shahriaree, 1983; Patel, 1978) may become inflamed from repetitive trauma.

Cartilage is composed of collagen, a proteoglycan gel, a few cells, and 60% to 80% water. It has no blood or lymphatic supply and therefore has a limited capacity for repair and regeneration (Mow, Roth, & Armstrong, 1980). Once damage occurs, often from abnormal wear because of some incongruity in opposing joint surfaces, there is no mechanism by which the cartilage can repair itself. This occurs, for example, when there is trauma to the patella resulting in softening and fibrillation of the articular cartilage of the patella (chondromalacia patella).

In contrast to cartilage, bone has great power to repair itself. In fact, the strength of bone is dependent on the forces placed on it, provided the forces are not greater than the mechanical strength of the bone, which would cause fracture. In running, repetitive forces on bone trigger increased remodeling in which resorption may outpace formation, resulting in the inability of bone to withstand the cumulative effect of multiple submaximal loads. The result is a stress fracture. Various factors come into play in this scheme, including the amplitude, frequency, and number of repetitions of the load, as well as the reparative ability of the bone.

Two biomechanical theories have evolved regarding the cause of stress fractures in athletes. One, put forth by Nordin and Frankel (1980), is that muscles fatigue during continuous strenuous activity, causing them to be less able to absorb energy; therefore, abnormally high loads are transmitted to bone. The other theory expounded by Stanitski, McMaster, and Scranton, (1978) is that the repetitive forces of the muscles at their insertion in bone overload the bone and cause stress fractures. The forces acting on bone during loco-motion are complex (Lanyon, Hampson, Goodship, & Shaw, 1975). Perhaps both mechanisms of overload are appropriate explanations in given circum-stances and anatomical locations. More biomechanical data are needed regarding the specific forces acting on bone before the mechanism underlying stress fractures becomes clear.

Vessels and nerves are two other tissues that may occasionally become compromised in runners because of repetitive stress. Compartment syndromes have recently been described by a number of authors (Logan, Rorabeck, & Castle, 1983; Martens, Backaret, Vermaut, & Mulier, 1984; Mubarek, Owen, Garfin, & Hargens, 1978; Veith, Matsen, & Newell, 1980). The compartment syndromes occur when pressures within the muscular compartments of the lower leg rise to a level that compromises vascular supply. "Effort thrombosis" of the deep veins of the calf has also been reported (Harvey, 1978). A variety of nerve-related problems can occur in runners including Morton's neuroma, nerve entrapments that sometimes affect the calcaneal or posterior tibial nerves, and sciatica, either from lumbar disc disease or occasionally from pressure secondary to spasm of the piriformis muscle.

Sex Differences in Injury Rates

Because of the problems mentioned earlier regarding the accurate reporting of injury rates among runners, it may be of benefit to explore differences in injuries among other groups to determine whether women are at increased risk of developing overuse injuries in running. Studies reporting injury rates for female military recruits and cadets at the service academies provide some insight into the differences in injuries between the sexes (Cox & Lenz, 1979, 1984; Kowal, 1980; Reinker & Ozburne, 1979). The majority of the injuries reported in these studies were similar to those encountered in distance running. Reinker and Ozburne (1979) found over twice the incidence of stress-related injuries in female than in male recruits. They could find no correlation between injury and height, weight, or age, but they did implicate poorly designed footwear for females in the etiology of some of the calcaneal and tibial stress fractures.

In another study of female recruits, Kowal (1980) found an incidence of reportable injury of 54%, which could be correlated with lack of conditioning, greater body weight and percentage body fat, and limited leg strength. In studies of the women midshipmen at the naval academy, Cox and Lenz (1979, 1984) concluded that, although women were treated three times more often for stress-related injuries than men, the incidence became less frequent as the women became accustomed to the more active life-style of the academy.

Other reports on the incidence of injury in men's and women's sports support the theory that higher rates of injury in women reported in the earlier studies were caused in part by lower levels of fitness and lack of conditioning (Clarke & Buckley, 1980; Garrick & Requa, 1978; Whiteside, 1980). As women became more active and more competitive in sports, their level of conditioning improved and their rates of injury approached those of men in similar sports.

Data on sex differences in running-related injuries are scarce. We must rely primarily on reports in the literature of specific injuries and the sex distribution of the patients that are reported. These data are, of course, susceptible to a variety of sampling errors and therefore must be interpreted cautiously. Clement, et al. (1981) provided fairly comprehensive data regarding sex differences in running injuries. They found similar patterns of injury in anatomical locations, but the incidence of specific conditions differed between the sexes. Of the 10 most common injuries in their series, Achilles peritendinitis and patellar tendinitis occurred at least twice as often in men, while tibial stress syndrome was about 1-1/2 times more frequent in women. Despite the belief that the wider female pelvis predisposes women to more patellofemoral problems, they did not find a significant difference in the incidence of patellofemoral pain. It was the most common injury in both sexes, occurring in 24% of the men and 27% of the women.

Reports on patellofemoral pain must be evaluated before they are compared, because different terms and definitions have been used to describe problems associated with the patellofemoral joint. Chondromalacia patella, a term describing softening of the articular cartilage on the undersurface of the patella, should not be confused with patellofemoral pain syndrome or patellofemoral stress syndrome, both of which are descriptive terms and do not necessarily imply softening of the cartilage.

Despite the problems with terminology, it is interesting to note other studies have failed to find an increased incidence of patellofemoral problems in women. Levine (1979) stated: ''While chondromalacia patella occurs at a two-to-one predominance in women in the general population, men outnumber women when only athletes are studied.'' In a prospective study of 100 athletes with the diagnosis of chondromalacia patella, men outnumbered women three to two (DeHaven, Dolan, & Mayer, 1979). Subluxation, another condition of the patellofemoral joint, was studied retrospectively by Henry and Crosland (1979), who found an equal ratio of men to women.

There is concern that stress fractures are occurring more frequently in women, especially stress fractures of the femoral neck and pubic ramus. Ozburn and Nichols reported that 67 out of 70 cases of pubic ramus stress fracture or adductor insertion stress reaction in military trainees occurred in women. In a study of runners, Pavlov, Nelson, Warren, Torg, and Burstein (1982) reported 9 out of 11 of their patients with pubic ramus stress fractures were women. In these two studies, the only etiologic factor that could be implicated in the cause of the fractures was overstriding, identified by Ozburn and Nichols as a result of female recruits trying to keep up with their taller male counterparts on marches. Female runners have also been found to have longer stride lengths relative to height and leg length than males (Nelson, Brooks, & Pike, 1977), possibly supporting the theory that overstriding contributes to pubic ramus stress fracture. The shape of the female pelvis was not believed by Pavlov, et al. to be an etiologic factor.

Whether stress fractures in general occur more frequently in females is more difficult to assess. Protzman and Griffs (1977) reported a 10-times greater incidence of stress fracture among female recruits. Taunton, Clement, and Webber (1981) reported a series of 62 runners treated for stress fractures. Thirty-seven (60%) were women. Other reports of runners appear to have at least equal numbers of females sustaining stress fractures (Roub et al., 1979). Stress fractures have been reported in almost every bone in the lower extremity. In some of the less commonly affected bones, the numbers reported are small, and conclusions regarding sex distribution would be dangerous. Some specific fractures, however, may occur less often in women. In a recent review of stress fractures of the tarsal navicular, only 2 of 19 patients were female (Torg et al., 1982). Iliac crest apophysitis and stress fracture in adolescents is also reported less frequently in females (Clancy & Foltz, 1976; Fernbach & Wilkinson, 1981).

If indeed stress fractures do occur more frequently in females, the causes of the increased incidence may be difficult to sort out. In addition to differences in anatomy, biomechanics, levels of fitness, and training regimens that must be identified, there may also be physiologic factors to be taken into account. Another chapter of this publication points out that a relatively high percentage of female endurance athletes are amenorrheic, and it has been recently documented that amenorrheic athletes have decreased bone mineral content in the lumbar vertebrae compared with their eumenorrheic counterparts (Drinkwater et al., 1984; Cann, Martin, Genant, & Jaffe, 1984). How and if these findings relate to the incidence of stress fracture in female athletes has not been determined, but it is tempting to speculate that there may be a relationship, especially in areas (such as the femoral neck) that are predominantly trabecular bone. The mechanism that governs bone mineral content and leads to lower values in the amenorrheic athletes is not known, but it is thought to relate to lower estrogen levels in women with exercise-associated amenorrhea. It has been demonstrated that physical activity may help prevent loss of bone mass in postmenopausal women (Smith, Reddan, & Smith, 1981; Krolner, Toft, Nielsen, & Tondevold, 1983; Aloia, Cohn, Ostuni, Cane, & Ellis, 1978). Also, male athletes have higher regional bone mass than sedentary controls (Aloia, Cohn, Babu, Abesamis, Kalici, & Ellis, 1978; Dalen & Olsson, 1974; Nilsson & Westlin, 1971). It appears that the exercise stimulus in the amenorrheic athlete is not sufficient to overcome the estrogen deficiency, at least in the lumbar spine. Both studies of amenorrheic athletes found no difference between the amenorrheic and eumenorrheic groups in the density of cortical bone at the wrist. More data are needed to determine the bone mineral content at other sites. Perhaps those areas that have the most stress maintain bone mass. Only further research will answer these questions.

It is apparent from the above discussion that no comprehensive data are available regarding sex differences in injury rates related to running. A variety of factors make it difficult to draw conclusions. Differences in fitness and training levels appear to be major causes of apparent sex-related differences, but other factors including anatomy, biomechanics, and physiology must be assessed as well.

Treatment

Treatment of the overuse injuries is first concerned with rest of the injured area, which in most cases can be accomplished by relative rest: merely reducing the activity that caused the injury while allowing any activity that does not exacerbate the condition. In some instances, however, the use of crutches or casting may be necessary. Inflammation is reduced and healing is promoted with anti-inflammatory drugs and a variety of physical therapy modalities such as ice, heat, and ultrasound. Finally, the cause of the overuse injury should be identified and corrected. In most cases the cause is a training error that can be dealt with by modifying the training program. Anatomical factors can be corrected with physical therapy to increase strength or flexibility, changes in shoes, or orthotics. Rarely is surgical intervention necessary to correct anatomical factors or to repair damage caused by overuse.

Summary

Most injuries in running are overuse injuries caused by repetitive trauma. The major cause of these injuries is training errors, although other extrinsic and some anatomical factors are often implicated. Injuries are common in runners of both sexes, although there are some indications that women may have a higher overall incidence of injury. Injury patterns are similar, but women appear to have a higher incidence of shin splints and stress fractures and a lower incidence of certain types of tendinitis. Treatment is aimed at rest, anti-inflammatory measures, and identification and correction of the cause of injury.

Further information is needed in many areas to more accurately determine the incidence and etiologic factors related to running. Greater knowledge may enable us to prevent rather than merely treat overuse injuries.

References

Aloia, J.F., Cohn, S.H., Ostuni, J.A., Cane, R., & Ellis, K. (1978). Prevention of involutional bone loss by exercise. *Annals of Internal Medicine,* **89,** 356-358.

Aloia, J.F., Cohn, S.H., Babu, T., Abesamis, C., Kalici, N., & Ellis, K. (1978). Skeletal mass and body composition in marathon runners. *Metabolism,* **27,** 1793-1796.

Brody, D.M. (1980). Running injuries. *Ciba Clinical Symposia,* **32,** 1-36.

Buchbinder, M.R., Napora, N.J., & Biggs, E.W. (1979). The relationship of abnormal pronation to chondromalacia of the patella in distance runners. *Journal of the American Podiatry Association,* **69,** 159-162.

Cann, C.E., Martin, M.C., Genant, H.K., & Jaffe, R.B. (1984). Decreased spinal mineral content in amenorrheic women. *Journal of the American Medical Association,* **251,** 626-629.

Clancy, W.G., & Foltz, A.S. (1976). Iliac apophysitis and stress fractures in adolescent runners. *The American Journal of Sports Medicine,* **4,** 214-218.

Clarke, K.C., & Buckley, W.E. (1980). Women's injuries in collegiate sports. *The American Journal of Sports Medicine,* **8,** 187-191.

Clement, D.B., Taunton, J.E., Smart, G.W., & McNicol, K.L. (1981). A survey of overuse running injuries. *The Physician and Sportsmedicine,* **9,** 47-58.

Clement, D.B., Taunton, J.E., & Smart, G.W. (1984). Achilles tendinitis and peritendinitis: Etiology and treatment. *The American Journal of Sports Medicine,* **12,** 179-184.

Cox, J.S., & Lenz, H.W. (1979). Women in sports: The naval academy experience. *The American Journal of Sports Medicine,* **7,** 355-357.

Cox, J.S., & Lenz, H.W. (1984). Women midshipmen in sports. *The American Journal of Sports Medicine,* **12,** 241-243.

Dalen, N., & Olsson, K.E. (1974). Bone mineral content and physical activity. *Acta Orthopedica Scandinavica,* **45,** 170-174.

D'Ambrosia, R.D., Zelis, R.F., Chuinard, R.G., & Wilmore, J. (1977). Interstitial pressure measurements in the anterior and posterior compartments in athletes with shinsplints. *The American Journal of Sports Medicine,* **5,** 127-131.

DeHaven, K.E., Dolan, W.A., & Mayer, P.J. (1979). Chondromalacia patellae in athletes. *The American Journal of Sports Medicine,* **7,** 5-11.

Drinkwater, B.L., Nilson, K.L., Chestnut, C.H., Bremner, W.J., Shainholtz, S., & Southworth, M.B. (1984). Bone mineral content of amenorrheic and eumenorrheic athletes. *New England Journal of Medicine,* **311,** 277-281.

Fernbach, S.K., & Wilkinson, R.H. (1981). Avulsion injuries of the pelvis and proximal femur. *American Journal of Rheumatology, 137*, 581-584.

Fulkerson, J.P. (1982). Awareness of the retinaculum in evaluating patello-femoral pain. *The American Journal of Sports Medicine, 10*, 147-149.

Garrick, J., & Requa, R. (1978). Injuries in high school sports. *Pediatrics, 61*, 465-469.

Gross, R.H. (1983). Leg length discrepancy in marathon runners. *The American Journal of Sports Medicine, 11*, 121-124.

Hardaker, W.T., Whipple, T.L., & Bassett, F.H. (1980). Diagnosis and treatment of the plica syndrome of the knee. *The Journal of Bone and Joint Surgery, 62-A*, 221-225.

Harvey, J.S. (1978). Effort thrombosis in the lower extremity of a runner. *The American Journal of Sports Medicine, 6*, 400-402.

Henderson, J. (1977). First aid for the injured. *Runner's World, 12*, 32-36.

Henry, J.H., & Crosland, J.W. (1979). Conservative treatment of patello-femoral sublaxation. *The American Journal of Sports Medicine, 7*, 1214.

James, S.L., Bates, B.T., & Osternig, L.R. (1978). Injuries to runners. *The American Journal of Sports Medicine, 6*, 40-50.

Kowal, D.M. (1980). Nature and causes of injuries in women resulting from an endurance training program. *The American Journal of Sports Medicine, 8*, 265-269.

Krolner, B., Toft, B., Nielsen, S.P., & Tondevold, E. (1983). Physical exercise as prophylaxis against involutional vertebral bone loss: A controlled trial. *Clinical Science, 64*, 541-546.

Lanyon, L.E., Hampson, W.G.J., Goodship, A.E., & Shah, J.S. (1975). Bone deformation recorded in vivo from strain gauges attached to the human tibial shaft. *Acta Orthopedica Scandinavica, 46*, 256-268.

Levine, J. (1979). Chondromalacia patella. *The Physician and Sportsmedicine, 7*, 41-49.

Lilletvedt, J., Kreighbaum, E., & Phillips, R.L. (1979). Analysis of selected alignment of the lower extremity related to the shinsplint syndrome. *Journal of the American Podiatry Association, 69*, 211-217.

Lindenberg, G., Pinshaw, R., & Noakes, T.D. (1984). Iliotibial band friction syndrome in runners. *The Physician and Sportsmedicine, 12*, 118-130.

Logan, J.G., Rorabeck, C.H., & Castle, G.S.P. (1983). The measurement of dynamic compartment pressure during exercise. *The American Journal of Sports Medicine, 11*, 220-223.

Marshall, J.L., Johanson, N., Wickiewicz, T.L., Tischler, H.M., Koslin, B.L., Zeno, S., & Meyers, A. (1980). Joint looseness: a function of the person and the joint. *Medicine and Science in Sports and Exercise, 12*, 189-194.

Martens, M.A., Backaert, M., Vermaut, G., & Mulier, J.C. (1984). Chronic leg pain in athletes due to a recurrent compartment syndrome. *The American Journal of Sports Medicine, 12*, 148-151.

Mow, V.C., Roth, V., & Armstrong, C.G. (1980). Biomechanics of joint cartilage. In V.H. Frankel & M. Nordin (Eds.), *Basic Biomechanics of the Skeletal System.* (pp. 61-86), Philadelphia: Lea & Febiger.

Mubarek, S.J., Gould, R.N., Lee, Y.F., Schmidt, D.A., & Hargens, A.R. (1982). The medial tibial stress syndrome. *The American Journal of Sports Medicine,* **10,** 201-205.

Mubarek, S.J., Owen, C.A., Garfin, S., & Hargens, A.R. (1978). Acute exertional superficial posterior compartment syndrome. *The American Journal of Sports Medicine,* **6,** 287-290.

Nelson, R.C., Brooks, C.M., & Pike, N.L. (1977). Biomechanical comparison of male and female distance runners. In P. Milvy (Ed.), *The marathon. Physiological, medical, epidemiological, and psychological studies* (pp. 793-807). *Annals of the New York Academy of Sciences,* **Vol. 301.** New York: The New York Academy of Sciences.

Newell, S.G., & Bramwell, S.T. (1984). Overuse injuries to the knee in runners. *The Physician and Sportsmedicine,* **12,** 81-92.

Nilsson, B.E., & Westlin, N.E. (1971). Bone density in athletes. *Clinical Orthopedics and Related Research,* **77,** 179-182.

Noble, C.A. (1980). Iliotibial band friction syndrome in runners. *The American Journal of Sports Medicine,* **8,** 232-234.

Noble, H.B., Hajek, M.R., & Porter, M. (1982). Diagnosis and treatment of iliotibial band tightness in runners. *The Physician and Sportsmedicine,* **10,** 67-74.

Nordin, M., & Frankel, V.H. (1980). Biomechanics of whole bones and bone tissue. In V.H. Frankel & M. Nordin (Eds.), *Basic biomechanics of the skeletal system* (pp. 15-60), Philadelphia: Lea & Febiger.

Nottage, W.M., Sprague, N.F., Auerbach, B.J., & Shahriaree, H. (1983). The medial patellar plica syndrome. *The American Journal of Sports Medicine,* **11,** 211-214.

Ozburn, M.S., & Nichols, J.W. (1981). Pubic ramus and adductor insertion stress fractures in female basic trainees. *Military Medicine,* **146,** 332-334.

Pagliano, J., & Jackson, D. (1980). The ultimate study of running injuries. *Runner's World,* **15,** 42-50.

Patel, D. (1978). Arthroscopy of the plicae—synovial folds and their significance. *The American Journal of Sports Medicine,* **6,** 217-225.

Pavlov, H., Nelson, T.L., Warren, R.F., Torg, J.S., & Burstein, A.H. (1982). Stress fractures of the pubic ramus. *The Journal of Bone and Joint Surgery,* **64A,** 1020-1025.

Protzman, R.R., & Griffs, K.G. (1977). Stress fractures in men and women undergoing military training. *The Journal of Bone and Joint Surgery,* **59A,** 825.

Reinker, K.A., & Ozburne, S. (1979). A comparison of male and female orthopedic pathology in basic training. *Military Medicine,* **144,** 532-536.

Roub, L.W., Gumerman, L.W., Hanley, E.N., Clark, M.W., Goodman, M., & Herbert, D.L. (1979). Bone stress: A Radionucleotide imaging perspective. *Radiology, 132,* 431-438.

Roy, S. (1983). How I manage plantar fasciitis. *The Physician and Sportsmedicine, 11,* 127-130.

Smart, G.W., Taunton, J.E., & Clement, D.B. (1980). Achilles tendon disorders in runners—a review. *Medicine and Science in Sports and Exercise, 12,* 231-243.

Smith, E.L., Reddan, W., & Smith, P.E. (1981). Physical activity and calcium modalities for bone mineral increase in aged women. *Medicine and Science in Sports and Exercise, 13,* 60-64.

Stanish, W.D. (1984). Overuse injuries in athletes: A perspective. *Medicine and Science in Sports and Exercise, 16,* 1-7.

Stanitski, C.L., McMaster, J.H., & Scranton, P.E. (1978). On the nature of stress fractures. *The American Journal of Sports Medicine, 6,* 391-396.

Steadman, J.R. (1979). Nonoperative measures for patellofemoral problems. *The American Journal of Sports Medicine, 7,* 374-375

Sutker, A.N., Jackson, D.W., & Pagliano, J.W. (1981). Iliotibial band syndrome in distance runners. *The Physician and Sportsmedicine, 9,* 69-73.

Taunton, J.E., Clement, D.B., & McNicol, K. (1982). Plantar fasciitis in runners. *Canadian Journal of Applied Sports Sciences, 7,* 41-44.

Taunton, J.E., Clement, D.B., & Webber, D. (1981). Lower extremity stress fractures in athletes. *The Physician and Sportsmedicine, 9,* 77-86.

Torg, J.S., Pavlov, H., Cooley, L.H., Bryant, M.H., Arnoczky, S.P., Bergfeld, J., & Hunter, L.Y. (1982). Stress fractures of the tarsal navicular. *The Journal of Bone and Joint Surgery, 64-A,* 700-712.

Veith, R.G., Matsen, F.A., & Newell, S.G. (1980). Recurrent anterior compartment syndromes. *The Physician and Sportsmedicine, 8,* 80-88.

Viitasalo, J.T., & Kvist, M. (1983). Some biomechanical aspects of the foot and ankle in athletes with and without shinsplints. *The American Journal of Sports Medicine, 11,* 125-130.

Wells, C.L., & Plowman, S.A. (1983). Sexual differences in athletic performance: Biologic or behavioral? *The Physician and Sportsmedicine, 11,* 52-61.

Whiteside, P.A. (1980). Men's and women's injuries in comparable sports. *The Physician and Sportsmedicine, 8,* 130-140.

Wild, J.J., Franklin, T.D., & Woods, G.W. (1982). Patellar pain and quadriceps rehabilitation. *The American Journal of Sports Medicine, 10,* 12-15.

Witman, P.A., Melvin, M., & Nicholas, J.A. (1981). Common problems seen in a metropolitan sports injury clinic. *The Physician and Sportsmedicine, 9,* 105-108.

Index